INTRODUCTION
YOGA, SURFING, AND
THE FLOW STATE

You don't have a life, You are life.

—Eckhart Tolle

If you're reading this book, it's likely you are feeling drawn to yoga and/ or surfing for their powerful and transformational benefits. Perhaps you already practice one or the other and are intrigued to discover how the two can be combined for an even more potent effect. Often simply watching either of these movement art forms in action can invoke the feelings of bliss, joy, calm, relaxation, and ease. Both embody beauty and grace, and when mastered, both exemplify being in perfect harmony with nature, flowing as one with life.

When practiced individually, the impact can be completely transformational. When combined, the experience can change you on fundamental levels in ways that can only be understood by those who have ventured into the deep waters of either or both.

These elevated states of being are not easily attained in the modern world, which is ruled by technology, smartphones, and concrete. It is only through direct connection with the natural forces that you may come to know this power on an intimate and profound level. The result is more than incredible health, fitness, and inner peace. There is a spiritual aspect to the practice of yoga and surfing that can be likened to attending church, for those who are spiritually nourished by the gospel. Only instead of a church, the temple is the ocean and beach, and the music is the sound of the waves, birds, dolphins, whales, wind, and your own breath.

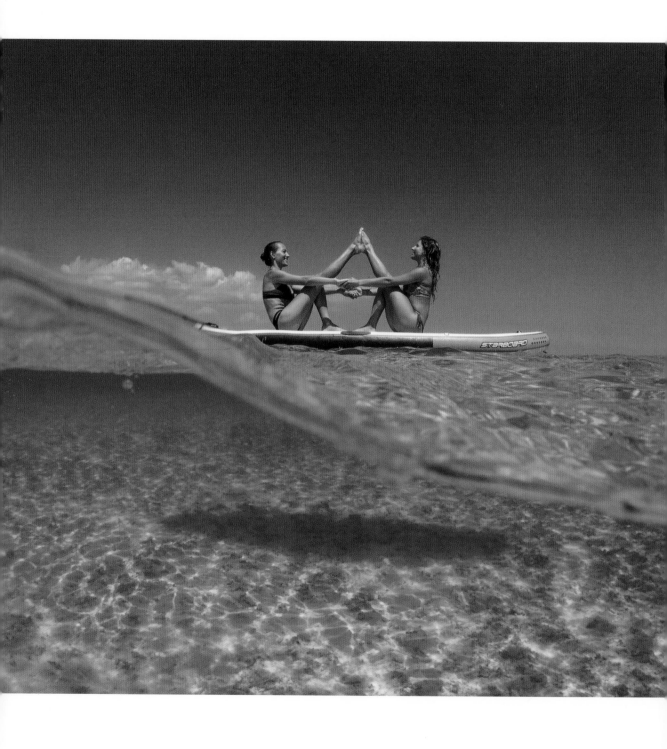

Understanding Yoga, Surfing, and the Flow State

Yoga is *union*. To be in union is to feel as one with the flow of life. This is the same objective for surfing, so we can naturally see how these go well together. The energy of flow is alluring and seductive. It is the very state of all that exists, as nothing is ever truly static in nature. All particles, molecules, cells, and living and nonliving beings in the universe exist in a constant state of flow. Even those objects that appear to be static, such as a rock or piece of metal, are in a subtle state of flow. Their molecules are simply much denser and vibrating close together, so that they appear to be solid.

Water is the only visible element where we can witness the energy of flow in its most apparent form. When a surfer enters the ocean, there is a relationship formed between the flow of the waves and the flow of consciousness that must be aligned for a successful ride to take place. The best surfers begin at a young age and practice relentlessly for years to master this art. The same is true for yogis. Some people are more naturally inclined toward this mastery from the beginning due to their essential nature given at birth, their environment, diet, or upbringing. Most people will need to train and practice to rise to a level of mastery of the flow. But when this happens, it can affect life on all levels.

When we master the flow state, we master our lives.

The flow state of consciousness is the realm where miracles, genius, outstanding creativity, and all mastery exist. It is pure potential without any blocks or barriers. In this state you feel the greatest sense of joy and happiness, as well as experience amazing health. Sickness, disease, pain, and injury do not exist in the flow state, or if they do, your awareness of how to heal and cure yourself becomes so clear, you rapidly move toward vibrant health. To enter the state of flow is also to heal yourself on the deepest level, as you align with your essential nature. This is the same essence as existence, so through this experience you become one with existence. It's not difficult to experience this for a moment or two, but to master sustaining it indefinitely is the aim of yoga. In yoga this state is often referred to as enlightenment, nirvana, or samadhi.

In the flow state you can access your innate or latent talents, without planning or preparation. There is no limit to the creative potential you may experience when you access this state; therefore, it is a way to experience the boundless and infinite nature of life itself.

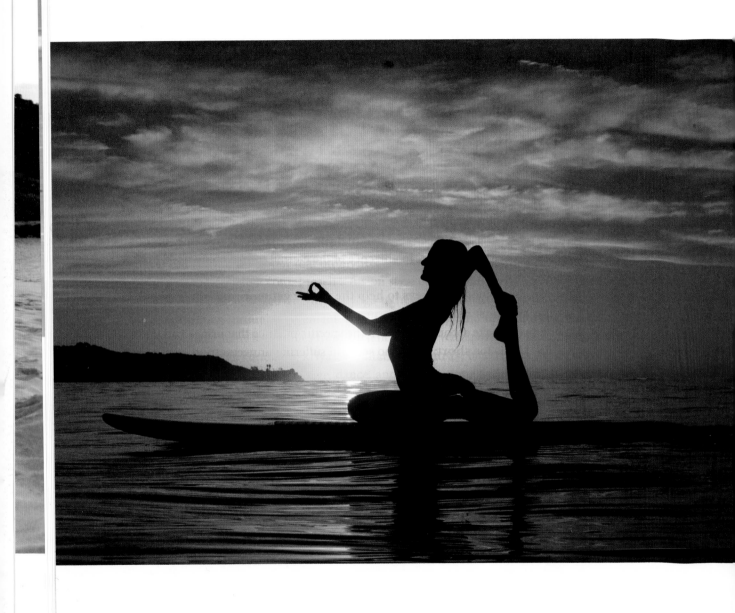

Understanding Yoga, Surfing, and the Flow State

Yoga is *union*. To be in union is to feel as one with the flow of life. This is the same objective for surfing, so we can naturally see how these go well together. The energy of flow is alluring and seductive. It is the very state of all that exists, as nothing is ever truly static in nature. All particles, molecules, cells, and living and nonliving beings in the universe exist in a constant state of flow. Even those objects that appear to be static, such as a rock or piece of metal, are in a subtle state of flow. Their molecules are simply much denser and vibrating close together, so that they appear to be solid.

Water is the only visible element where we can witness the energy of flow in its most apparent form. When a surfer enters the ocean, there is a relationship formed between the flow of the waves and the flow of consciousness that must be aligned for a successful ride to take place. The best surfers begin at a young age and practice relentlessly for years to master this art. The same is true for yogis. Some people are more naturally inclined toward this mastery from the beginning due to their essential nature given at birth, their environment, diet, or upbringing. Most people will need to train and practice to rise to a level of mastery of the flow. But when this happens, it can affect life on all levels.

When we master the flow state, we master our lives.

The flow state of consciousness is the realm where miracles, genius, outstanding creativity, and all mastery exist. It is pure potential without any blocks or barriers. In this state you feel the greatest sense of joy and happiness, as well as experience amazing health. Sickness, disease, pain, and injury do not exist in the flow state, or if they do, your awareness of how to heal and cure yourself becomes so clear, you rapidly move toward vibrant health. To enter the state of flow is also to heal yourself on the deepest level, as you align with your essential nature. This is the same essence as existence, so through this experience you become one with existence. It's not difficult to experience this for a moment or two, but to master sustaining it indefinitely is the aim of yoga. In yoga this state is often referred to as enlightenment, nirvana, or samadhi.

In the flow state you can access your innate or latent talents, without planning or preparation. There is no limit to the creative potential you may experience when you access this state; therefore, it is a way to experience the boundless and infinite nature of life itself.

Yoga and surfing teach, in overt and subtle ways, how to access the flow state of consciousness, and when combined, the practitioner can find themselves in an otherworldly experience. Beyond the incessant thoughts and confines of the mind, beyond the emotional turbulence and ups and downs of life, in a place that feels like infinite stillness, there is a realm often referred to as the void. The void is actually not empty, it is infinite flow. It is simply beyond thoughts, so it can feel like emptiness; however, it is actually the realm where everything exists in an infinite eternal flowing state of pure essence. This is the realm of the akasha, which in yoga is known as the realm of pure spirit.

As a yogi, a teacher, and a student of flow, I often see people entering the journey at various stages of mastery. In the beginning, it can feel somewhat awkward and can even be painful. This is true for all of life, as well as for yoga and surfing. Why? Because as the body-mind consciousness becomes attuned to a new way of being, old patterns and beliefs must die. When you lose mental focus and "check out" is when the tragic moment usually occurs.

It is in these moments that pain can be the greatest teacher. It can occur in yoga, when a student attempts a new pose or transition that is far beyond their current level and feels the anguish of tight or weak muscles, tendons, and ligaments and their apparent physical limitation. In surfing the same anguish may occur as the new surfer attempts a barrel wave only to become caught in its perilous grip and come crashing down upon a reef or some other potential hazard.

But if you ask a master surfer about these perils, you will get the same response every time: It's all part of the learning process. You have to go through it until you learn to become one with the ocean. And the yogis express the same sentiment. Except instead of becoming one with the liquid ocean, yogis aim to become one with the ocean of existence. If the promise is big enough, in this case mastering the flow and/or the wave, the price you have to pay often feels less steep.

Time and again you will see the novice surfer stand back up after a big fall, wipe off the blood from their rib cage, and paddle back out to give it another try. This is especially true for those surfers who have had a taste of the promise and reward at least a few times, so they will do whatever they can to grow, get better, or possibly just get their fix. After all, the natural high and exhilaration one experiences as a result of catching an epic wave, gliding across the water with seemingly effortless grace, can be addictive. Not to mention, simply being in the ocean is purifying and cleansing for the body, mind, and energy.

It is the same for yoga. Every yogi who has ever experienced even a taste of the feeling of being in the flow state, and the same natural high and euphoria that results from this, becomes hooked and a lifetime evangelist. Yoga is so miraculous because it doesn't only allow you to enter into this incredible state of consciousness, but it also has the power to heal the body and mind along the way.

To understand the divine union of yoga and surfing, we must first explore each individually, to show the power they offer when they stand alone.

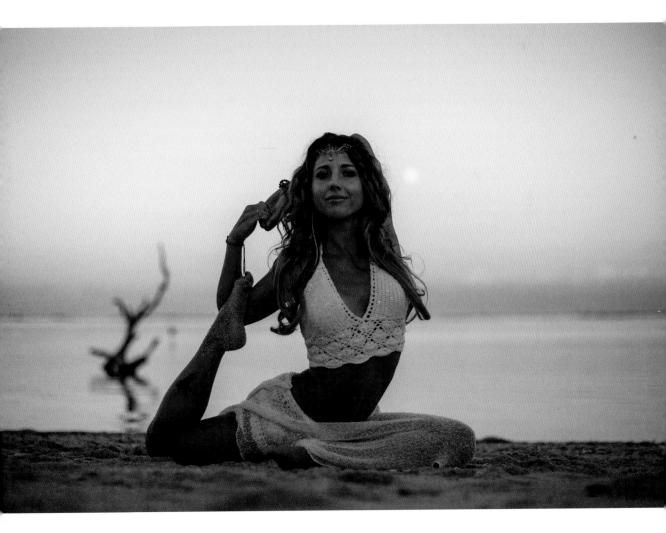

The Power of Yoga

There is now tremendous scientific research that shows that when yoga is practiced as a complementary regime along with other activities, the results of all other activities improve.

Why might this be?

Yoga, when taught and practiced properly, is meant to heal, balance, and restore the body and mind. It strengthens the areas that are weak, stretches the areas that are tight, and with consistency helps you to create a true sense of balance both physically and emotionally.

Yoga is a safe and powerful way to learn the art of flow. If taught properly, there is little chance for injury, and more commonly it will heal any aches, pains, or imbalances you might be experiencing in your body and life. The art of flow is most effectively taught in the vinyasa yoga style, although other styles of yoga can begin to teach this through both practice and theory, as they all start with the basic premise that the breath is your connection to life.

The more you practice yoga, the more attuned you become to the subtle essence of your spirit, which allows you to access the flow state naturally, as it is the state that transcends the mind's incessant thoughts.

Meditation, another aspect of the holistic science of yoga, can also teach you how to access the flow state. Although there are many forms and styles of meditation, it is also related to the guidance you have when embarking upon this journey. Just as the experience of learning to surf will be dramatically different for a surfer who learns at the North Shore in Hawaii from a pro or a surfer who learns in Miami Beach from a novice, for example, the methods and environment can truly make all the difference in one's experience. For those seeking the master level experience, it's always advisable to train with the masters. For all other intents, you can learn from the local yoga teacher at your health club and begin the journey just as well.

They say that when the student is ready, the teacher appears. In this book I will introduce you to the top surfing yoga masters in the world. It's an honor and privilege to learn from the masters, and you can trust that they will guide you in the right direction. These teachers not only master the flow state in yoga, but also master it on the waves. The practices they share in each chapter are those that work best for them and that they feel will most powerfully guide you on your way.

As the saying goes, "You can lead a horse to water, but you can't make him drink." In other words, you can read about yoga and how it may benefit you, but only through consistent practice will you achieve the greatest results. Yoga is a lifelong journey, and once you get started, just like surfing, you realize there really is no end.

There is a level of mastery you can attain and strive toward, but even as you reach that level you start to see there is always further to go. The path is deeper than the unexplored areas of the ocean and as wide and vast as the entire cosmic universe. There is an unending eternal, infinite unboundedness to the journey that can be both intimidating and alluring. As you access deeper realms of your own self-mastery and consciousness, you can also begin to grasp the infinite nature of existence itself.

All this and yoga will also make you feel really good. That same euphoric bliss-fulness that you feel when you catch an epic wave can become a steady and consistent vibration of your energy with regular yoga practice. Just as surfers tend to be easygoing and go with the flow, yoga can help to loosen up any rigidity or discontentment of the personality. There are practices for every need and desire, whether you want to simply become more flexible, release pain from your body, strengthen your core, or elevate your mood and energy. Yoga can do all this and so much more.

In this book, each practice that is offered has a specific intention. So feel free to use this book prescriptively. When you need to unwind, relieve stress, and relax, go with the practices in the tenth chapter. If you are seeking a more vigorous workout to empower your energy and strengthen your core, try chapter 3. You can choose to practice outside on the beach, on your surfboard or paddleboard on the water, or in the comfort of your home on a traditional yoga mat.

My intention is for you to use this book as a reference manual, coming back to it daily or as often as you can. Find the practices that work for you and feel free to share them with your friends and loved ones. Consistency is the key to your success, and self-mastery is closer than you know.

Best wishes to your incredible journey!

Love and blessings,

Tashrama

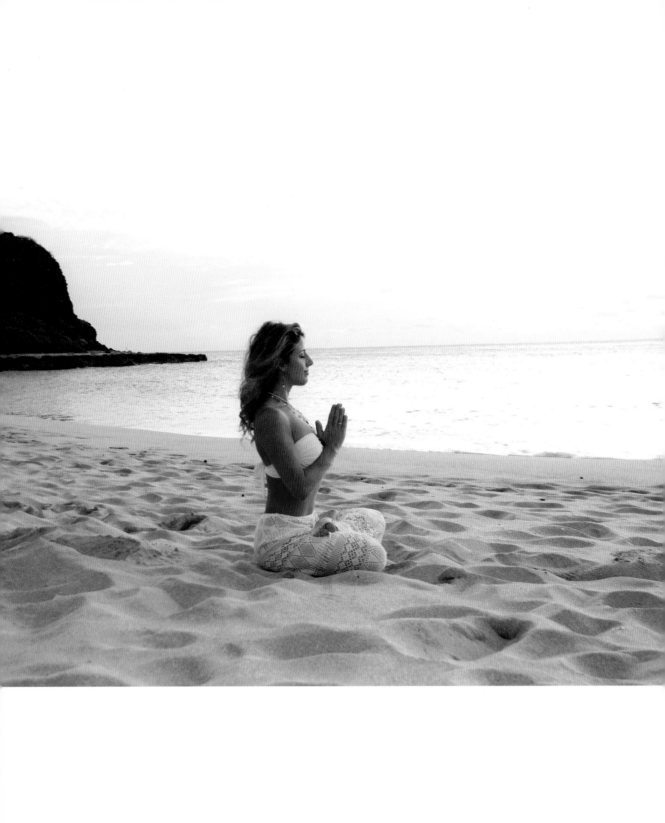

BEACH YOGA BLISS
Dashama Konah

My heart is open and I am living in harmony with life.
—*Dashama*

About Dashama

Dashama is an internationally known yoga teacher, author, speaker, producer, athlete, and happiness guru and the founder of the Global 30 Day Yoga Challenge, Perfect 10 Lifestyle, and Pranashama Yoga Institute. She is an innovator in the field of yoga, body-mind transformation, and healing, and has had the opportunity to speak at the United Nations and collaborate with Harvard University. She has been featured in the Wall Street Journal, Inc, Forbes, Cosmo, Vogue *and on* ABC, NBC, Fox, *and* Discovery Channel *and more. She has been sponsored by Starboard SUP, where she has a signature line of paddleboards, Nike, Puma, Vitamix, and GoPro. Her online video training courses reach over fifty million students worldwide and are in the top sellers list on Udemy, she is part of the Mindvalley Zenward yoga tribe, Jillian Michael's Fitfusion tribe on Broadband TV and ATT U-verse, and her YouTube videos have reached over thirteen million viewers.*

Dashama developed the Prasha Method system of healing after using these techniques to heal her own life and thousands of students around the world, both live and online. She teaches that the power of the mind is the greatest influence in your conscious evolution. Pranashama Yoga Institute offers 200- and 500-hour Yoga Alliance Approved Yoga Teacher Transformation Training Programs worldwide. Dashama has personally trained and certified hundreds of yoga teachers from the United States,

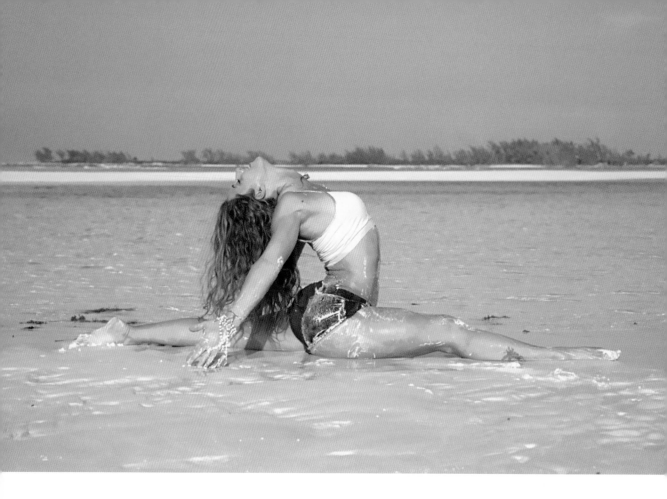

United Kingdom, Germany, Luxembourg, Italy, Finland, Norway, Russia, South Africa, Australia, New Zealand, Brazil, Colombia, Peru, Spain, Pakistan, Burma, New Caldonia, Canada, Mexico, and India. Learn more about Dashama's global yoga trainings at pranashama.com.

Dashama's signature trademarked 30 Day Yoga Challenge video training system is accessible for all levels and a perfect option to help you get started with a daily yoga, conscious living, and meditation practice from home. Learn more at 30dyc.com.

For free videos, meditation audios, and ebooks, visit Dashama's websites at dashama.com and pranashama.com, and join her global tribe of yoga lovers committed to making a positive impact in the world while living in the flow connected to the source of life.

Beach Yoga Bliss: Dashama's Practice for Health, Harmony, and Happiness

Yoga is for everyone. Regardless of your current state of balance, flexibility, or strength, the physical practice of yoga asanas can help you improve your current state and lead you toward a more harmonious experience in your body. You only get one body to live in this life, so it's essential to take great care of your temple.

The following yoga poses (aka asanas) are wonderful for creating an overall state of well-being. Once a level of proficiency has been achieved in each asana, you can begin moving toward fusing them together into a vinyasa sequence, connecting each pose with the flow of the breath for a calm, centered mind state.

In the beginning, yoga can feel uncomfortable and even painful in some ways, as you are made aware of the areas in your body that are tight, weak, and out of balance. With consistent practice, each of these issues can be resolved and your body will find its way back to its intrinsic equilibrium, which is a natural and state of harmony and perfect balanced health.

The asanas in this chapter target the major areas of the body that often become tight, weak, or out of balance from daily living. So these asanas can help tremendously whether you spend your days riding waves on a surfboard or answering emails at a computer desk.

To begin, find a quiet, peaceful, and inspiring place away from distraction to practice. If you can be outside, that's even better; being in nature and surrounded by the nourishing prana (energy) of Mother Earth is tremendously helpful to enhance your experience.

Before beginning the asanas, sit quietly for a few moments and begin to become grounded in your body and mind. Start to calm yourself and connect with your breath. As you inhale, feel your lungs expand and fill every cell of your body with prana, a cleansing and powerful life force energy. As you exhale, release any tension or stress from your body and mind.

1. Butterfly: All Levels

Starting in a seated position, bend both knees and bring the soles of your feet together. Press your knees toward the earth, externally rotating the hips and opening the soles of your feet toward the sky. With each breath relax your hips more toward the earth. If this is too challenging for you at first, you may wish to place a cushion, rolled-up towel, or block under your hips to elevate them above your knees. This will make this hip-opening pose more accessible until your hips loosen up. To deepen the stretch, fold for-

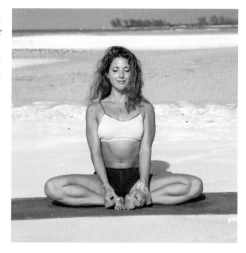

ward as you continue to press your knees toward the earth. Hold for 5–10 breaths at first, and progress until you can hold the pose for 30 seconds or over a minute. The longer you can hold each pose, the deeper you will go and the more progress you will make. Continue to breathe and enjoy the journey.

2. Cow Face/Gomukhasana Prayer: All Levels

Start seated with your knees bent and stacked on top of each other, as closely as possible If you need to put a cushion under your hip, it may help until your hips loosen up. Place your hands in prayer above your head to make this a centering meditative pose. When both hands are together, in prayer mudra, you invoke a deep heart connection; elevating this mudra above your head

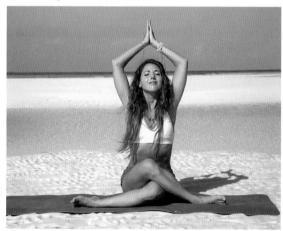

will raise this connection to an even diviner nature.

3. Seated Spinal Twist: All Levels

Start seated with your left knee bent and the left foot near your right hip, right leg crossed over left, right foot placed near the outer edge of your left thigh. As you inhale, sit up straight and lengthen your spine. As you exhale, twist your torso, placing your left elbow on the outside of your right knee and your right palm on the earth behind your back. Hold for 3 breaths and repeat on the other side. On each inhale, lengthen the spine; on each exhale, twist a little deeper.

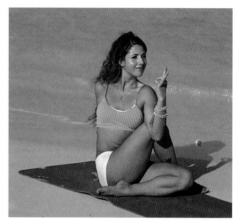

4. Mermaid: Level 2/3

Start with your left knee bent and forward and your right leg extended back while keeping both hips as "square" or flat toward the earth as possible. If this is not possible yet, you can support the alignment by placing a block, cushion, or rolled-up towel under your left hip to keep the balance between both hips. Start with a few simple breaths in the basic hip opening pose, also known as pigeon, which is the foundation of mermaid.

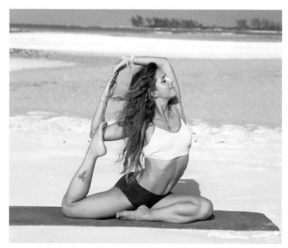

From there, if your shoulders and hips are open enough to allow you to, bend your right knee (back leg) and reach your right hand back for the right ankle, opening the right quad and hip flexors. If it is possible for you to maintain your spinal alignment, reach your left hand back to bind with the right. Hold for a few breaths and then release and repeat on the other side.

5. Low Crescent Lunge: All Levels

Start in a low lunge, with your right foot forward, right knee at a 90-degree angle and left leg extended back behind you with the knee on the earth and the top of the foot planted firmly to stabilize. Engage your core to stabilize as you reach your arms above your head. Palms can be in prayer, or interlace the fingers to feel more centered. Radiate your hips forward and lift your heart to the sky. Hold for 3–5 breaths and repeat on the other side.

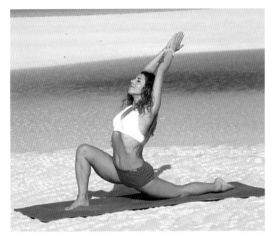

6. Low Crescent Lunge: Level 2

Start the same as low crescent lunge. If your spine feels open and flexible, start to arch your upper back, keeping the tailbone tucked under to lengthen the lumbar spine, as you lift your heart and gently arch back. Relax your arms down by your sides. Place your hand on the front knee or feel free to place your hands anywhere you feel will stabilize you to be able to hold this pose for at least 3 breaths. Be sure to do both sides.

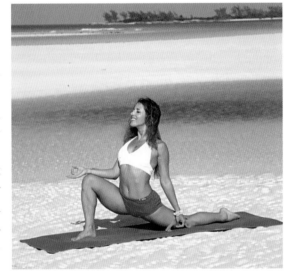

7. Upward-Facing Dog: All Levels

Starting on your belly, place your palms beneath your shoulders and begin to lift your chest toward the sky while pressing firmly into the tops of your feet. Lifting your knees and thighs, engage your core and lengthen your spine as you arch your upper back into a strong yet gentle backbend. Hold for a few breaths and slowly lower. Repeat 3 times to build strength and flexibility.

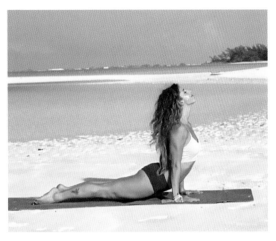

8. Bow Pose: All Levels

Lying on your belly, bend your knees and reach back with both hands toward each ankle. With your shoulders internally rotating so your thumbs are pointing down, reach back and grasp each ankle and start to lift your toes toward the sky. As your toes reach toward the sky, use your arm and back strength to lift your shoulders up and back, coming into a nice backbend. Turn your gaze up toward the sky as you root down through your belly and pelvic area. Hold for 5 breaths, release, and repeat 3 times. After your final bow pose in the sequence, go into child's pose to counterbalance your spine.

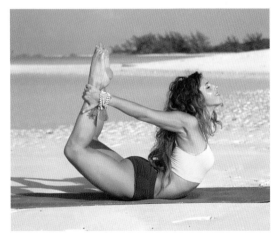

9. Crow: Level 2

This core-strengthening arm balance pose is the foundation for most other arm balances. To begin, place your palms shoulder distance apart on the earth, spread your fingers, and grip the earth slightly to create a strong foundation. Engage your core and bandhas (yogic energy locks) to draw the energy in and up (imagine a magnet is pulling you toward the sky from your upper back as you root down through your palms). Place your knees on your upper triceps, one at a time, then lift your feet up and point your toes back. Look forward and shift some weight forward to create equilibrium.

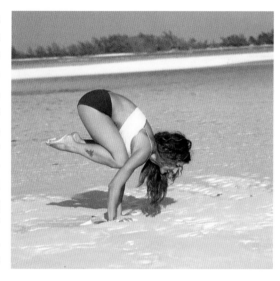

10. Goddess: All Levels

Start with your legs wider than hip distance apart, feet turned out to the sides, knees above your ankles, legs spread as wide as they can go. Sink your hips as low as you can, engaging your glutes and thighs while maintaining a firm foundation with proper form. Lengthen your spine from the lower back by tucking the tailbone under a bit and lifting your heart and the crown of your head toward the sky. Hold for 5–10 breaths and then straighten your legs. Repeat 3 times.

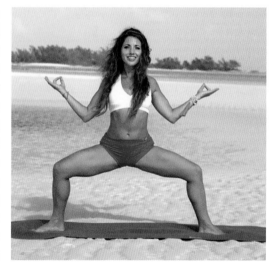

11. Goddess Toe Balance: Level 2

Start the same way as described for goddess, but lift the heels as high as you can to balance on your toes. This requires more stability, so engage your core and bandhas, lengthen your spine, sink your hips down, and spread your knees. Place your palms in a prayer position above your head to raise the energy upward. Focus should be across from you, on something that is not moving. Hold for 3–5 breaths and repeat 3 times. As you gain strength and balance over time, try to hold longer to continue to improve.

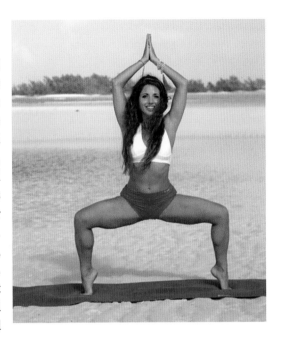

12. Tree with Hawaiian Prayer Mudra: All Levels

Shift your weight to your right foot, spread your toes, lift your arches, and engage the right leg as you lift your left foot to place the sole of the foot on the ankle, inner calf, or thigh of the standing/base leg. Lift the kneecap of the base leg to engage the quadriceps, engage your core, lengthen your spine, and reach your arms out and up with your palms facing the sky. Feel the flow of prana/energy rise from the earth toward the sky and then ground down from the sky to the earth. Keep your focus on something that is steady and not moving. Hold for a few breaths, then switch legs and repeat on the other side.

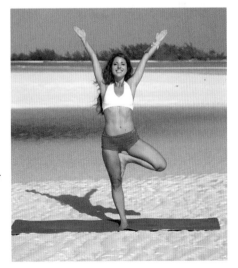

13. Standing Hand to Foot: Level 2

Start as if you're going into tree pose, with your right foot firmly rooted on the earth and quads engaged to activate your foundation. Bend your left knee and reach your left hand "peace fingers: index, middle, and thumb" to clasp the big toe on the left foot. Extend your left leg as straight as possible as you drop the left hip down parallel to the right hip and the ground. Place your right hand on your right hip and lengthen your spine, lifting the crown of your head to the sky, shoulders back, drishti (focus point) straight ahead. Hold for 3–5 breaths and repeat on the other side.

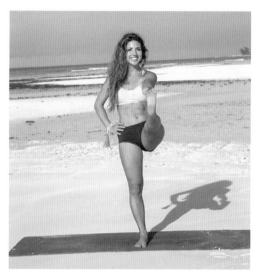

14. High Standing Crescent Lunge: All Levels

Start with your left leg forward, left foot firmly planted on the earth, left knee bent, right leg extended behind you, right knee lifted, stabilizing on your right toes, both hips squared to the front of the mat. Tuck your tailbone slightly as you lengthen your spine and lift your chest toward the sky. Pull in your lower belly and engage your bandhas and core muscles. Reach your arms up by your ears, placing your palms together either in prayer or fire mudra, fingers interlaced. Hold for 5 breaths and repeat on the other side.

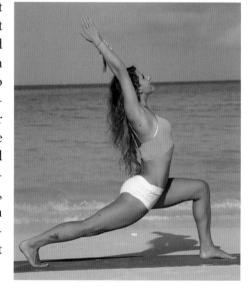

15. Warrior 1 with Eagle Arms: Level 2

Start similar to high standing lunge, except turn your back foot flat with the toes rotated forward 45 degrees. Root down through the back heel and draw the front hip back to square the hips forward toward the front of the mat. With a long spine and strong core, wind your arms around each other, right arm under, left arm on top, placing your palms together into a prayer position in front of your face. Press your elbows away from your chest and your fingertips toward the sky to open the upper back and shoulders. Breathe deeply for 3–5 breaths and repeat on the other side.

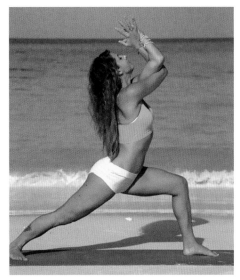

Guided Meditation for Inner Peace and Joy

Start seated in gomukhasana (cow face) with arms extended above in Hawaiian prayer.

We call this Hawaiian prayer position, with arms open to the sky and heart lifted. In this open-armed position, which is a form of a mudra or kriya, you open yourself to receive, which is to invoke the feminine receptive energy of the divine in your practice. If this seated position is too uncomfortable, then sit with your legs crossed in any comfortable position you can hold for a few minutes. Just keep your spine erect and

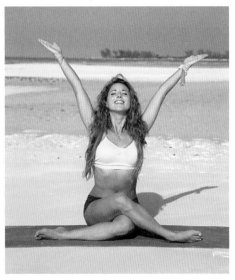

straight, as that is the essential aspect to have the best experience in all seated meditation postures.

You can keep your arms extended or, if that is too challenging, place your palms on your heart or rest your palms facing up on your legs or knees during this meditation. The intention of this meditation is to connect with your natural state of inner peace and joy, which will raise your overall vibration and state of being.

Start with your eyes closed and begin to connect with your breath. As you inhale, simply observe how the flow of air enters the nostrils, and connect with the pause between the inhale and the exhale before releasing the breath. Connect with a steady rhythm of breath and feel any tension or stress melting away from your body. As you release deeper and deeper into a state of mental relaxation, begin to draw your awareness to your heart center. Feel the breath expand the lungs, expanding your heart and filling your body with a feeling of peace. If any thoughts of your life come into your mind, step outside of these thoughts and witness them as a silent observer. See that all is in divine and perfect order. See that life is on your side. See that everything is always working out for you. Know that everything is exactly as it is supposed to be.

Now we will invoke the Hawaiian prayer of forgiveness: Ho'oponopono.

In the Hawaiian tradition there is a very powerful prayer to create harmony and heal all relations. It's simple, and anyone can benefit from this practice. The traditional kahunas, who were the Hawaiian shaman s, passed this down for many generations, and now we can invoke the miracles in our own lives through this simple yet profound teaching.

There are four parts to the prayers, each addressing an aspect of human relations and invoking healing into these aspects. You can repeat this prayer just one time or as many times as you desire, even addressing the prayer toward a specific person, situation, or circumstance you wish to heal in your life or in the world at large. The power of prayer is immense, so be ready for miracles! As you clear the energy within yourself toward all your relations, you will notice an immediate shift of your own vibration.

You can do this daily or as often as you like. I even know people who do this all day every day as a walking mantra meditation, simply repeating the prayer to create a positive energy field surrounding them everywhere they go. Just do what works for you and enjoy the experience. Feel free to reach out to me to share your experience. I'd love to hear about it!

The Ho'oponopono Prayer
I love you. (Love)
I am sorry. (Compassion)
Please forgive me. (Forgiveness)
Thank you. (Gratitude)

Feel free to modify this slightly, by adding the name of who you are addressing with the prayer or even directing it toward yourself. For example:

I love you, mother.
I am sorry, mother.
Please forgive me, mother.
Thank you, mother.

In my practice I have gone on to expand it even further to include specifics. For example:

I love you, mother.
I am sorry, for the pain you experienced in the final years of your life.
Please forgive me, for anything I may have done or not done, I tried my best to help you heal.
Thank you, for giving me life and for showing me nonattachment so early in life.

This is just one example, but I hope you get the idea. The more you can feel the prayer in your heart and connect with the energy and emotions of love, compassion, forgiveness, and gratitude, the more powerful and miraculous this prayer and meditation experience becomes. Try doing this daily for eleven or thirty days and see if you can notice a shift in your energy, relationships, and way of relating to the world.

With consistent practice of this prayer and meditation, you will notice an uplifting feeling of inner peace and joy in your heart, mind, and life. As you gain this deep clarity of energy within you, it will ripple out to everything and everyone around you. In this way, you are being the change that will shift the world.

Like a domino effect, as each one of us on earth takes personal responsibility for our energy and state of being, we positively raise the vibration for all humanity.

Enjoy the journey and be blessed!

Sat Nam and Namaste,
Dashama

FalconGuides Interview: Get to Know Dashama Konah

Q. Who or what brought you into yoga to begin with? How did you get started and what got you hooked?

A. My parents were both into yoga before I was born. My father told me his first girlfriend, when he was twenty years old, was a yoga teacher, and he met Swami Muktananda in New York City when he was in his early twenties. My mother was a very spiritual, psychic, shamanic type of woman. She was born and raised in the Black Hills of South Dakota, and she frequently meditated and had altars everywhere in our house when I was a young girl. We lived in a rural area, and I'd spend hours outside in nature meditating and reading books. When we went to visit my grandparents, who lived at the beach in Boca Raton, Florida, I fell in love and got hooked on the ocean. Now that I'm older I can see how both yoga and the ocean have been instrumental in my life from the very start. As a young girl, my parents taught me some basic postures like headstand, full wheel pose, mermaid, and the splits. They tried to keep it fun for me back then. That was my first introduction to yoga.

My mother lost her mind when I was seven, and I was sent to live in foster homes for many years after that; it was a difficult time for me growing up. Later, in middle and high school I was involved in many sports and was always elected to be the stretch leader for the teams. So I guess I was teaching yoga from a young age, which was healing for me. Back then it wasn't known as yoga, we just called it stretching. Many of the kids didn't like it because it was painful after a long running practice, but I made them do it. It helped everyone's performance on the team, so the coaches were also supportive. I was hooked from day one, since it felt like an essential and necessary part of life. Like breathing and eating, I feel stretching and moving my body in fluid motion have been absolutely essential to my evolution, to feeling good, and to shifting energy and emotions that arise, as they often do.

Q. What about surfing? How did that happen? Who, what, when, where, and why did you start and what has that journey been like?

A. I started surfing very young, but back then I was just bodysurfing or my other favoriate way, which is to surf beneath and through the waves. I tried surfing on a surfboard for the first time back in 2007, in Nosara, Costa Rica. I was a guest teacher at my friend Leslie Glickman's yoga retreat, and for one of the excursions we got to try surfing lessons with the local Tico pro surfers. That was a challenging time for me. I recall the surfboard seemed ten feet long and was very heavy; I couldn't carry it and had to drag it down to the water. I had used some BullFrog sunblock and when my face got wet, the toxins from that product leaked into my eyes and I felt like I was going blind. After a few hours my torso and belly were rashed up from the board. I didn't give up, though, and kept trying to surf that day. I remember how beautiful it was out on the ocean, and the instructor was a great coach. He gave me great confidence and I did catch a few waves that first day. I came away feeling accomplished, but I had only just touched the feeling of the flow state through surfing for a few seconds. It gave me even greater respect for the incredible pro surfers who can catch and surf massive waves all day. It's a physically challenging and incredibly beautiful sport.

Since then I've surfed a bit in many oceans, including in Bali, Hawaii, Florida, California, and Spain. I got more into paddleboard yoga in 2009 and fell in love with that, since you can do it when there are no waves. we have another option called SUP surfing that is becoming popular now, where you can surf on a paddleboard designed for surfing waves, but you have the paddle with you so you stay standing the whole time. Laird Hamilton had originally made SUP surfing famous with his big wave surfing in Hawaii. I like that a bit better than getting up and down all the time, but just being on the ocean is always the best feeling in the world for me.

Q. Can you describe your first or most transcendent experience with yoga? Anything that made you experience the flow state we are talking about in this book?

A. My first yoga teacher training, back in 2005, ushered me into that experience in the most unexpected way. I had always been a hyperactive person with loads of energy. In India they have a word for it—pitta—and another word they use is rajasic, which is to have too much energy and not know what to do with it. During my first yoga teacher training, to balance the doshas, they required us to stop eating all spices, even garlic, onions, and all pepper, for example. We were allowed to eat only satvic foods, which means pure, simple, and holy foods. I had been addicted to caffeine before that, so this alone started to change my life. Then, since it was a traditional style of yoga, called sivananda yoga, they required us to take a five-minute savasana meditation between each pose. This was a huge breakthrough for me, since I had not been able to meditate much in my life, due to my hyperactivity. As a teenager I even had a hyperactive thyroid disorder, which for years made me feel as if I were burning alive from the inside out. That later resulted in the removal of my thyroid, so I had faced this hyperactive energy most of my life.

During the training we had to meditate between each pose in the yoga classes every day for ten weeks and listen to their very calming music, which felt like it put me into a trance state. I later learned that the music was mantra music, holy music from India. I remember specifically one song, the "Devi Mantra," changed my life. As I went through the yoga classes and workshops each day for the training and laid there in the meditation pose in between each asana, many times I would cry as the layers of old pain and stuck energy were being peeled away. After a few weeks I started to notice a real change in my mind state. The mental fluctuations were calming down, and I was starting to experience stillness inside for the first time. We chanted mantras and meditated in silence each morning from 6:00 to 7:00 a.m. for those ten weeks, and that also changed my life. I didn't really understand how it was working at the time, but all of these subtle things we were doing were changing my life. It changed my brain, my energy, and my whole perspective on life, and I was never the same again.

I remember walking along the beach one afternoon during those ten weeks of training and realizing there had been absolutely no thoughts inside my mind for several hours. I felt interconnected with everything. The ocean, the tide, the whole universe, and I were one, and I only heard the low hum of the mantra "Om" in the back of my consciousness. It brought a stillness to my body and heart and a sense of liberation. It felt as if I had merged completely with eternity, that time had stopped, yet there was a knowing that I was present in that experience, and my observer witness consciousness was aware that this was a turning point in my life. Before that teacher training I was just practicing yoga a few times a week as part of my fitness routine along with weight training, kickboxing, running, and many other modalities. After that experience on the beach, something changed inside me, and I fully committed my life to spreading the miracle of yoga.

Q. What about surfing? Was there an experience that stands out more than the rest, and can you describe it in words? Where were you?

A. As a young girl, I always felt like a fish in the water. Even though I wasn't surfing on a surfboard back then, we would bodysurf for hours in and under the ocean waves. I remember one experience when I was around eight years old, at the beach house where my grandparents lived in Boca Raton. I had been surfing under the waves for hours and hours when suddenly a massive manta ray swam directly under me, about five to ten feet away. In that moment everything stopped, and the universe and all of existence went to complete stillness as I encountered this massive and majestic divine creature. Later in life I researched the meaning of the manta ray spirit animal, which, according to spirit animal science, symbolizes the flow state. That made so much sense, and since then I have experienced the same feeling in the presence of wild dolphins and whales in the wild ocean while swimming, paddleboarding, underwater yoga, surfing, or bodysurfing. The combination of ocean, majestic sea animals, and surfing, which immediately invokes a feeling of complete awe and wonder, the feeling of oneness and interconnection with all that exists, is the flow state in its most primal form and experience for me.

Q. Are there specific places on earth where you feel most connected to this energy or flow state of consciousness, whether you are practicing yoga, surfing, both, or just being?

A. I feel a strong connection to places with dense jungle and tropical rainforests that meet the ocean. Some of my favorite vortexes on earth are Bali, Hawaii, and Costa Rica. In these environments I feel many layers of stress start to melt away and I can more easily access the flow state, as it is the pure essence in the vortex of these natural environments. Anywhere I am in the ocean, I feel it, but even some oceans and beaches on earth carry more powerful energy than others. Hawaii is one of the top places for me in the world. There is a very unique energy the natives say comes from the goddess Pele, the goddess of the volcano that gave birth to the islands. Her power comes from a very deep place, the core magma lava of earth, and you can actually feel this when you are in Hawaii and especially while swimming or surfing in the ocean there. When there are waves, this gives the ocean even greater power and energy. And combined with pristine fresh air, sunshine, and even some wind, it's very invigorating and enlivening.

Q. Where and how did you start out in yoga? What was your first introduction to the practice and how do you suggest people start if they are considering getting into yoga? What is your favorite style to practice? Do you teach yoga? If so, what style?

A. As I mentioned earlier, my parents introduced me to yoga at an early age. I'm so grateful for that, since it really helped me through the hard times over my lifetime. It took me many years to discover the depth of the practice and path of yoga, however, since it is not obvious at first how deep yoga can take you, by simply seeing some photos or taking a class at the gym. I suggest people who are seeking to start a yoga practice try a variety of styles to discover what resonates best with their needs, goals, and energy. There are literally hundreds of styles, and they are all very different. I suggest you try local classes, online classes, workshops, or retreats. I have online classes, workshops, and even online yoga teacher trainings as well as the live trainings and retreats that I lead worldwide. You can learn more about that on my website at pranashama.com or at my personal site at dashama.com. I teach a fusion style called Pranashama yoga, which is an open system based on vinyasa yoga to help people access the flow state of consciousness through movement, meditation energy, and breath. Pranashama incorporates many techniques from ancient lineages with powerful life-changing practices such as kundalini, kriyas, meditation, mantras, bhakti, yin yoga, shivananda, tantra, thai yoga massage, dance, and even qi gong and tai chi. The open system allows for the evolution of the practice as we are always learning, growing, and expanding our understanding and awareness of the infinite nature of source energy that streams to us and through us at all times. Through yoga, we are able to access that energy, channel it to heal, restore, awaken, and transcend anything that is not in alignment and harmony with our true and divine nature.

Q. Do you feel a beginner can access the feeling of the flow state either in yoga or surfing, or would you say it's more of an advanced practice that they can work their way up to with consistent dedicated practice?

A. Anyone can tap into the flow state at any stage of development or life experience, such as how Eckhart Tolle or Sadhguru both explained they simply fell into the experience of the now and decided to stay there permanently. Although those are rare and powerful examples, based on one's prior experience with music, movement, breath work, spiritual practices, and other factors, it may be easier to access this state with some practice over time. I like to think of it like a lotus flower unfolding and blossoming. It takes time for all of the petals to unfold. To access the flow state, you must dedicate time and energy toward the inner experience and train your mind to concentrate and focus, to let go of thoughts, and to simply be present with whatever is arising in each moment. It's a state of divine surrender into presence. Some people are born with this ability; it may take many years for others. It's not so much a skill as it is a surrendering. We must surrender all that we think we know, since all thoughts are generally just blocking the flow. The true flow state is beyond thoughts. The miracle is that when we let go of all rational mind activity, we can actually access an infinite well of understanding, wisdom, and knowledge that comes directly from the source of life itself. As long as we realize we are just channels for the universe to work and flow through us, we can truly be the embodiment of the miraculous, beyond anything we could have possibly dreamed. Human potential is far beyond anything our minds can fathom. To access the flow state is to tap into the realm beyond the thinking mind and connect to the wisdom and intelligence of the eternal source of life itself.

Q. Can you share some tips/keys to help the reader get more out of the practice of yoga and/or surfing?
A. I suggest you make a commitment to the specific practice that brings you the greatest joy. Life is too short; there's no sense in suffering unnecessarily.

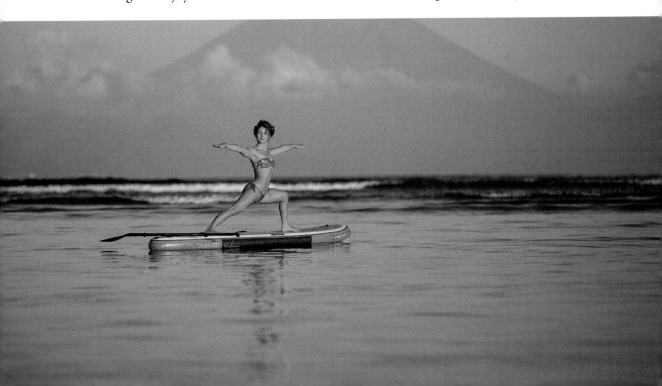

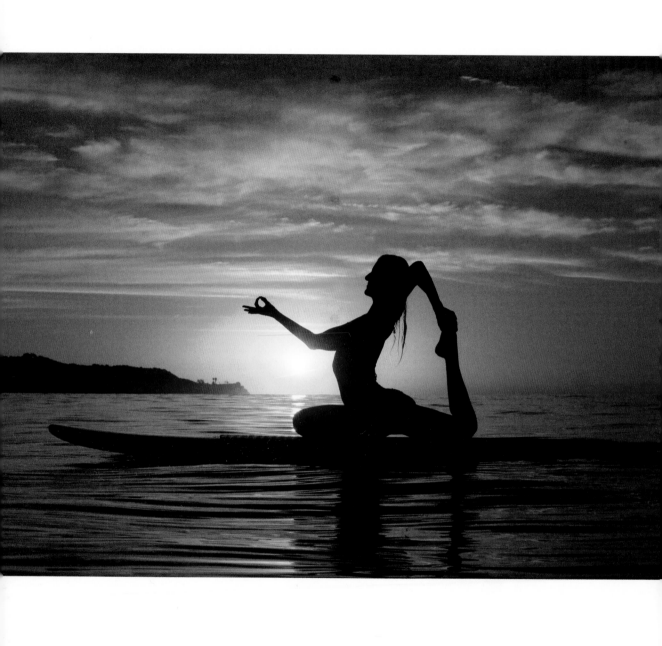

EMBODY THE FLOW
Shiva Rea

Life is change. Learn to surf.

—*Swami Satchidananda*

About Shiva

Shiva Rea offers yoga and surf retreats around the world as part of Yoga Adventures as well as a Surf Yoga Soul *DVD (Acacia) and online practices on Yogaalchemy.com. As the founder of Prana Vinyasa and Samudra Global School for Living Yoga, the Global Mala Project, and Be-A-Light Solar Lantern Project, she supports yoga for all as conscious evolution around the globe. Visit her at pranavinyasaflow.com.*

Shiva's Prana Flow Namaskar for Embodying Fluidity and Strength for the Waves of Life

I offer here a short version of a prana flow namaskar (salutations) that is not the typical "shoulder opening" sequence we think of for surfing. (I have a yoga and surf DVD called *Surf Yoga Soul* that has a lot of strength and flexibility sequences specific to surfing.) This particular flow opens your side body, inner and outer hips, and spine in a flowing sequence that allows you to be responsive to change. Most of the forty namaskars of prana vinyasa are offered in a mandala, or circle, to open up our awareness 360 degrees. Enjoy embodying the flow.

1. Tadasana

Step with your feet hip-width apart and join your hands together at your center. Move into a flow state as you begin ujjayi breathing—the sound of the ocean being drawn on the back of your throat to create a meditative anchor in which to breathe fully in the present moment. Shift your weight forward and back as if you were on a surfboard, to feel your pelvis centered over your feet and your heart and crown of the head in alignment. Anchor your tailbone toward the earth and feel your lower belly rising upward to support your spine.

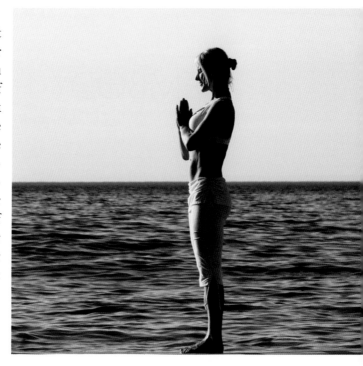

2. Standing Anahatasana (Heart-Opening Pose)

Inhale and open your arms wide. Exhale, placing hands to sacrum, rooting down. Inhale, rising up from your feet and lower belly to lengthen and strengthen your spine. Arch back slowly through your upper back.

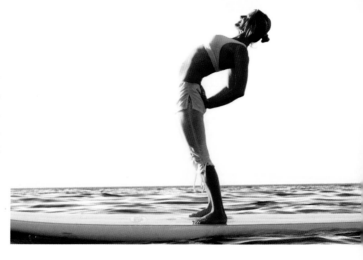

3. Uttanasana (Forward Bend)

Exhale as you hinge at your pelvis, slowly leading with your heart as you fold into a forward bend. Breathe into your hamstrings and keep reaching through your heart to massage your spine. If needed, bend your knees slightly but keep your heart open instead of rounded.

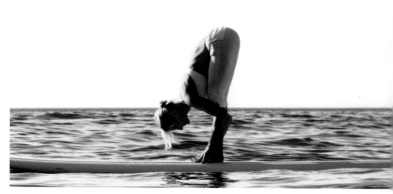

4. Anjenayasana (High Lunge)

On an exhalation, step your left foot back into a high lunge with your front knee over your front ankle and your back heel pressing away.

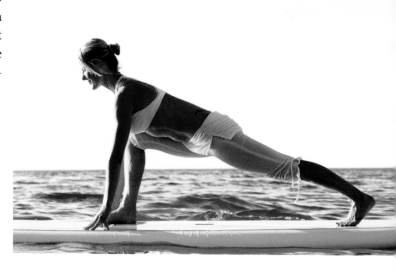

5. Prana Flow Lunge I

Inhale and draw your right arm overhead as you turn both feet clockwise. Your front foot is at a right angle; your back foot is in side plank. Open your side body and outer hips, and feel the fluidity within stability in this prana flow variation of lunge.

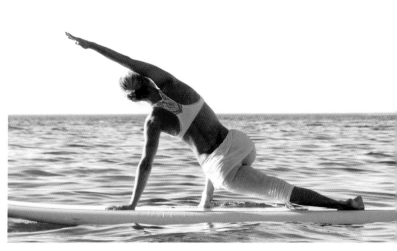

6. Prana Flow Lunge II

Exhale and reach your right hand toward your back foot with your chest open, shoulders level, and legs activated. Move between prana flow lunge I and II two more times.

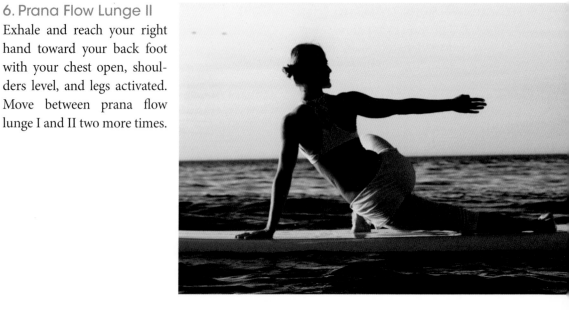

7. Sahaja Ardha Malasana (Spontaneous Flowing Half Squat)

Exhale as you turn your whole body counterclockwise until you are standing with your feet wide and parallel to one another. Inhale, bend your right knee and extend your left leg, keeping the spine long. Exhale, gathering energy from your inner legs to your pelvic floor. Inhale and shift to the other side with the same awareness. Now flow back and forth twice more, sweeping your arms and torso in a spontaneous flow, like seaweed in the ocean.

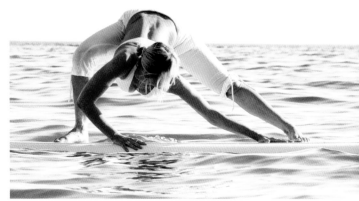

8. Anjenayasana (High Lunge)

Turn toward your left leg to again come into a high lunge, right leg back, with your front knee over the ankle, radiating through the back heel.

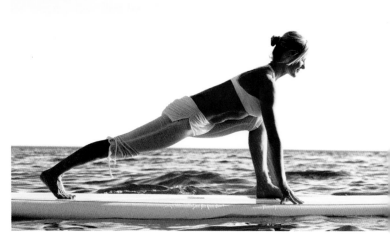

9. Prana Flow Lunge I

Inhale and draw your left arm overhead as you turn both feet clockwise. Your front foot is at a right angle; your back foot is in side plank. Open your side body and outer hips, and feel the fluidity within stability.

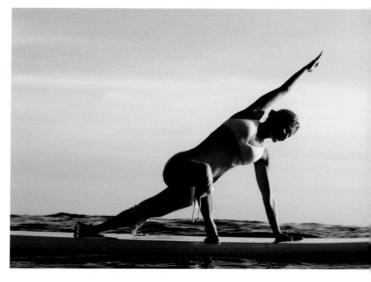

10. Prana Flow Lunge II

Exhale and reach your left hand toward your back foot with your chest open, shoulders level, and legs activated. Move between prana flow lunge I and II two more times.

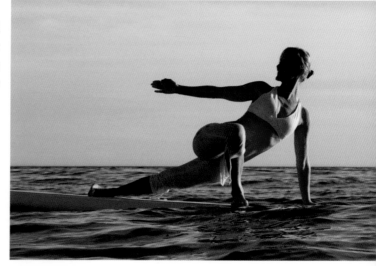

11. Dandasana (Staff)

Inhale and step your left leg back into dandasana with your hands under your shoulders, your core activated, and a long line of energy from crown to tailbone to heels.

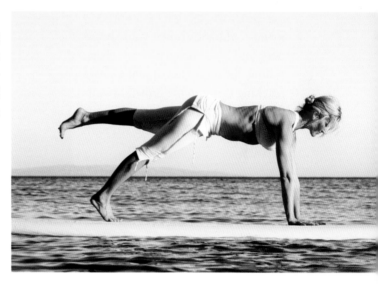

12. Anahatasana (Heart-Opening Asana)

Exhale and lower both knees to the floor, lower belly engaged. Walk your hands out in front of you, shoulder-width apart, and release your heart to the earth. Rest for several breaths, then slide forward and lower all the way down.

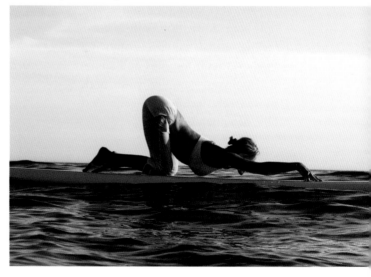

13. Bhujangasana (Cobra)

Bring your hands under your shoulders and rise through your chest, rolling through the shoulders and reaching through the crown of your head. Stretch back through your legs to your toes. Feel the strength whether you are low or high.

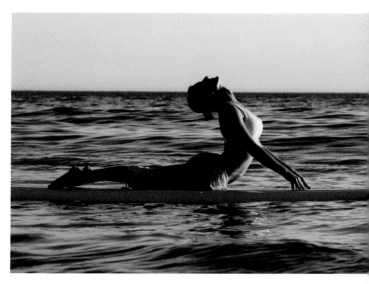

14. Adho Mukha Svanananda (Bliss-Filled Downward Dog)

Exhale, curl your toes under, and flow into down dog with a lunar feeling. Pedal the heels, moving freely through the hips and spine. Release your jaw, let your neck move freely, feel the self-generated bliss of a liberated dog.

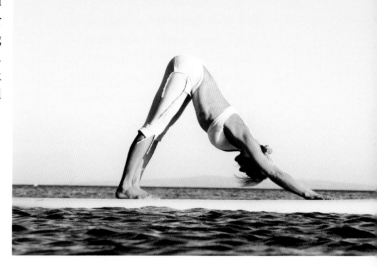

15. Uttanasana

Walk your hands back to your feet, "hands on the earth." Lift through the hips and curl over your feet, straightening your legs and releasing your spine toward the earth. Take your hands to hips and massage down the backs of your legs, softening into the forward bend.

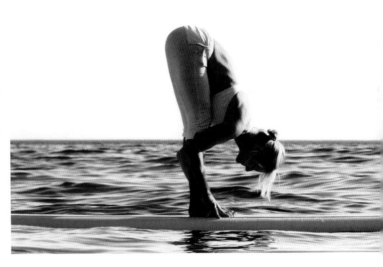

16. Standing Anahatasana

Rise to standing, hands to the base of the spine. Feet rooted into the earth, draw energy up the legs and along the spine to arch through your upper back.

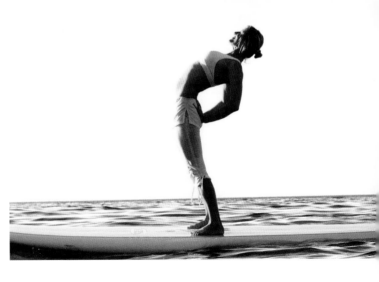

17. Tadasana

Take a moment and center yourself, and either dive down again for 35 more rounds, or be ready to surf—or surf the waves of life.

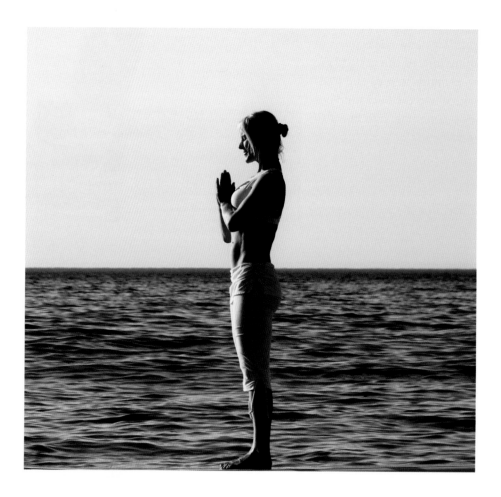

FalconGuides Interview: Get to Know Shiva Rea

Q. Who or what brought you into yoga to begin with? How did you get started and what got you hooked?

A. I was born in Hermosa Beach, California. The beach was literally my front yard and created the greatest influence in the unfolding of my life. The imprint of the waves—the pulse of life—was always part of me. My father was an avid surfer and named me Shiva after the "Lord of the Dancing Universe" that he experienced while being with the ocean waves. So the seed was planted for my journey for both surfing and yoga. We moved to Berkeley when I was four, so it was not until later in life that surfing awakened the connection to the flow experience. Now everything has come full circle, and I am a surfing yogini dedicated to embodying the flow on the water, in yoga, and in life.

Q. What about surfing? How did that happen? Who, what, when, where, and why did you start and what has that journey been like?

A. I didn't seriously start surfing until my late thirties when I moved a mile from Sunset and PCH in Pacific Palisades in a year of amazing waves. It was the first time in my life surfing year-round in a drop-it-all-for-the-swell rhythm. I started including surfing lessons in my yoga teacher trainings in Southern California and then moved into surfing and yoga retreats. Now I also love kayaking waves when the surf is low. There is nothing like the direct contact with the living ocean, to be in harmony with the changing currents. No wave is the same. It takes courage to drop into a breaking wave, willing to fall and be churned for the possibility of that moment when time slows down as you ride a glassy wave, feeling the power moving you and moving in harmony with its energy.

Q. Can you describe your first or most transcendent experience with yoga? Anything that made you experience the flow state we are talking about in this book?

A. I always remember my first yoga experience as being initiated on my own at age fourteen from a book I found in the library to learn more about my name. I followed the instructions exactly as I went into the hip opener pose, upavista konasana. It was the simple process of being tuned in to my breath and the sensations I was experiencing that totally transformed my state of being. My worries dissolved into a profound sense of being and connectedness. It launched my

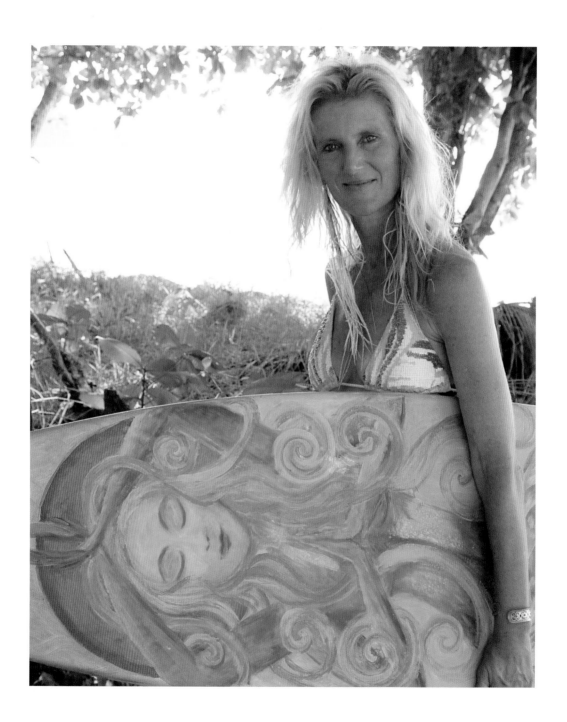

journey, and now my focus is on leading vinyasa as movement meditation—surfing the flow of embodied breath awareness.

Q. Can you name your favorite surf break and where that is? What about for new surfers, is there a best place to learn in your opinion? Did you start with lessons or just go out and take the waves on? Is your family into surfing or were you a pioneer in your family?

A. My favorite surf break is in Nosara, Costa Rica, where both newbies and big wave riders can enjoy the same long stretch of amazing, consistent waves with the jungle coming up right to the beach. I also love the North Shore of Kauai, and my favorite local surf break is County Line in Malibu.

Q. Where and how did you start out in yoga? What was your first introduction to the practice and how do you suggest people start if they are considering getting into yoga? What is your favorite style to practice? Do you teach yoga? If so, what style?

A. So after that seed was awakened when I was fourteen, I started to practice a Tantric-based mantra meditation system and then later become an Ashtanga practitioner while studying world arts and cultures at UCLA. I ended up living around the world from the age of seventeen, in East and West Africa, India, Nepal, Bali, and Jamaica, where I studied movement as meditation and ritual and its role in cultural change. Now after twenty-five years of teaching, I offer Prana Vinyasa Flow around the world in retreats, teacher immersions, festivals, and large-scale activations including sacred activism for seva, or service.

Shiva's Tips for Yoga and Surfing Success

Your breath is your greatest teacher when you simply contemplate the experience that you are being "breathed." The flow state begins when you let go of pushing the breath and experience the inner intelligence of your life force. You can feel that in movement, in an asana, and when you sit or walk. That "just rightness." You can feel it and let your breath/life-force teach you from the very beginning. In a prana vinyasa practice, we say you are simply "surfing" the flow of the breath or "slow dancing with your breath." If you have either surfed or slow danced this week, then you know that feeling.

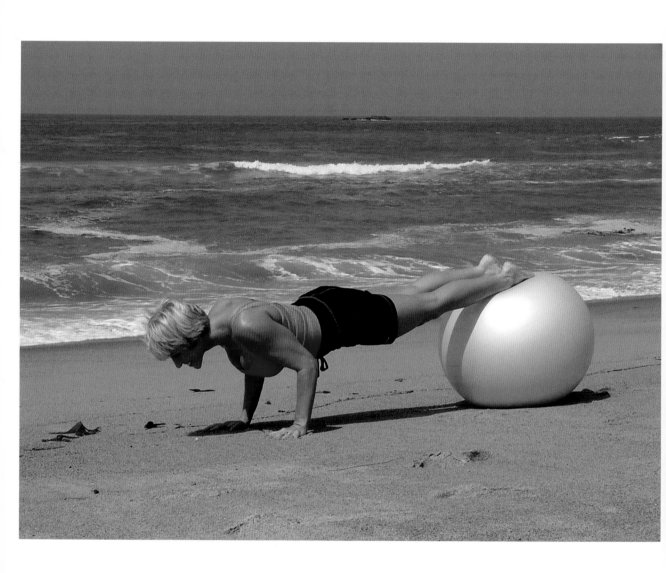

YOGA FOR SURFERS PIONEER
Peggy Hall

The moment of being on a wave is so fleeting—yet so thrilling—that you want to experience it again and again, no matter how many waves you catch! Like surfing, yoga gives you a glimpse into what it is to be in that place of utter freedom—completely outside of the boundaries of time, constraints, obligations, and expectations—just powerful, alive, open, and free!

—*Peggy Hall*

About Peggy

Called a "legend" by Surfer *magazine, Peggy Hall is an avid surfer and certified yoga instructor who is recognized as the pioneer of the modern surf and yoga movement. Since 2002, her best-selling* Yoga for Surfers *instructional DVD series has transformed the lives of tens of thousands of surfers around the world.*

Peggy is also a leading wellness expert, author, speaker, and radio and television personality who shares her passion for Living Swell® with her signature natural health and beauty products.

Peggy first discovered yoga when she began surfing in her mid-thirties. Her intention was to heal her chronic shoulder tendinitis from years of competitive swimming. Not only did her shoulder heal, but her surfing improved dramatically. Looking for a surf-specific yoga video but finding nothing like that existed, Peggy put her passions together and created the world's first Yoga for Surfers *instructional video series. Peggy also runs* Yoga for Surfers *Teacher Training Programs to prepare instructors to teach surf-specific yoga at retreats, camps, and diverse locations around the world.*

Known for her enthusiastic and inspiring teaching style, Peggy's clear, encouraging instruction makes even the most demanding poses accessible to all, and her radiant energy is a testament to the life-enhancing benefits of yoga.

In addition to her passions for yoga, surfing, and healthy living, Peggy is a fierce animal welfare advocate involved in education and community outreach through her organization, CompassionforAll.org, which works to save the lives of neglected and abandoned animals that otherwise would have no hope.

Peggy's Tips for Yoga and Surfing Success

As surfers, we thrive on the energy of the ocean. We feel totally alive when we connect to the power of the waves and awaken the essence of our being. We want nothing more than to stay in the water as long as possible and to surf with as much energy and endurance as we can. We want to catch more waves and surf them better than ever. We want to experience the transforming energy that only a soul-cleansing surf can offer.

As surfers, yoga helps us achieve all that and more.

Yoga

1. At its essence, yoga is freedom. Focus less on executing a perfect pose and more on experiencing yourself in the pose. Where can you release, relax, and let go even more?

2. Move in a way that feels good to your body. Avoid forcing or straining, which can create more tension in your mind and muscles. Allow your body to open in its own time.

3. Let go of the notion of good and bad or right and wrong. There's no such thing as being "good" at yoga—it's all good when you're simply breathing and staying calm and aware. Let go of any judgment or criticism about yourself and the pose.

Surfing

1. Befriend the ocean. Learn how to read the waves, the weather, the conditions. Realize that certain days you'll be on the beach instead of in the water. When you're not surfing, practice yoga to work on your strength, endurance, flexibility, balance, lung capacity, and mental focus.

2. Warm up before paddling out. Spend about five to seven minutes doing some easy stretches (get ideas at yogaforsurfers.com). Focus on conscious breathing throughout your surf session.

3. Open yourself to the totality of the surfing experience. Take note of the weather, the water temperature, the sea life, all of creation. It's not the wave count; it's about making each wave count through conscious awareness and endless gratitude. Enjoy your special time in the water basking in the beauty of creation and the power of life itself, whether or not you catch any waves!

Peggy's Fluid Power Practice for a Quicker Pop-Up

Getting a quicker pop-up is something every surfer wants. That's because a quick pop-up is what's needed to get into the wave faster, so more of the wave can be ridden and more pure stoke can result!

A quick pop-up requires three things:

1. Powerful shoulder and arm muscles (specifically, pectorals and triceps)

2. A strong core, including hip flexors (to bring the legs up on the board, front foot under the torso)

3. Coordination and balance (so the legs come up in a fluid, powerful, and coordinated manner, conserving energy)

The following consists of innovative variations on classical yoga poses:

1. Flowing Warrior 2 Combined with Triangle (Warm-Up)

With legs wide and arms extended, inhale as you bend your front knee to come into warrior 2; exhale as you straighten your leg. Inhale and move into triangle, with both legs straight; exhale and return to standing. Repeat 3 times per side.

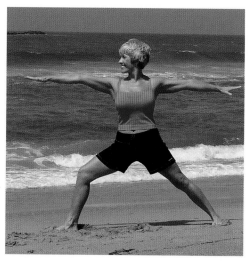

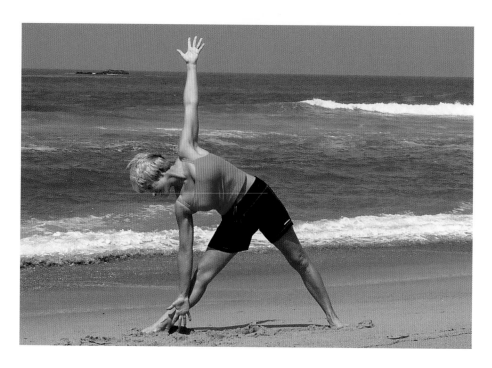

Option: To work your shoulders, arms, and core, return to warrior 2, wrap the top arm behind your back and extend the bottom arm, pressing against your inner thigh. Hold for 3 breaths. Repeat sequence on other side.

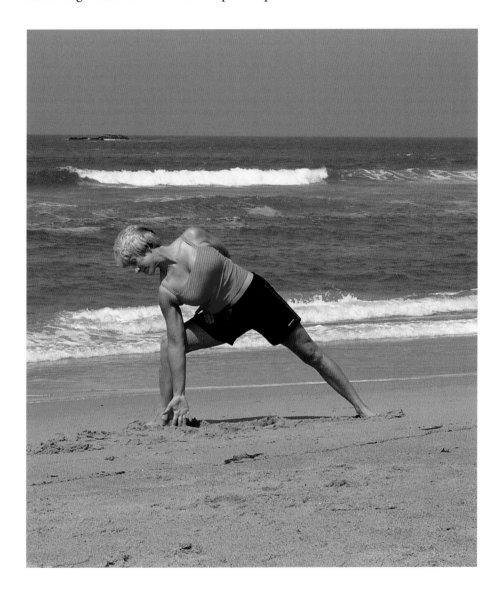

2. Stability Ball Plank/Push-Up (Strength)

Using a stability ball, come into a push-up position, with the tops of your feet on the ball. This is a variation of chaturanga, a type of yoga push-up.

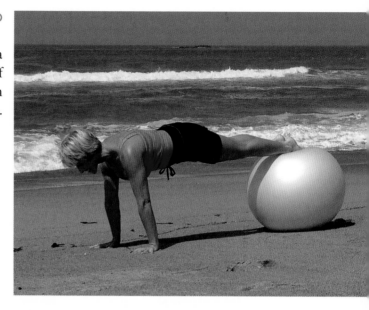

Inhale and bend your elbows, hugging the upper arms to your chest. This position directly mimics the arm position on your surfboard for your pop-up. Exhale as you press back up, powerfully, to starting position.

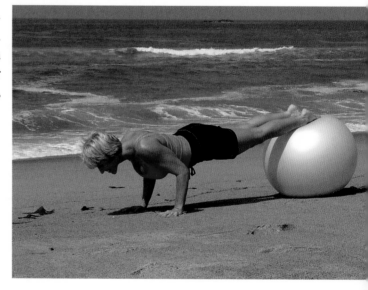

With your toes on the ball, engage your abdomen and lift your hips high, rolling the ball toward you for a hip lift. This activates the psoas, the hip flexor muscle responsible for bringing your legs under your torso for a quick pop-up. Roll the ball back to starting position and repeat the push-up sequence and hip lift 58 times.

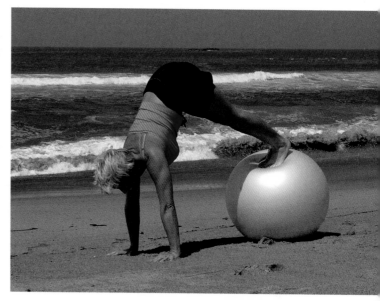

Option: Repeat the sequence with one leg lifted for more of a challenge. Doing these moves on a stability ball helps you develop balance and coordination.

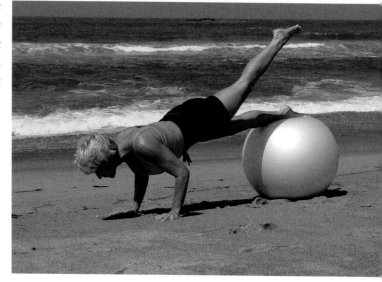

3. Warrior 3 with Triceps Extension (Strength and Balance)

This variation on warrior 3 builds core strength and balance while developing the back of the upper arm (triceps) for greater power when you push off the deck of your surfboard on the pop-up.

Use a pair of hand weights (5–8 pounds or your desired amount of resistance). Balance on one leg, extending your other leg behind you, strong and active, with the knee facing the ground. Extend your arms toward the ground, palms facing each other.

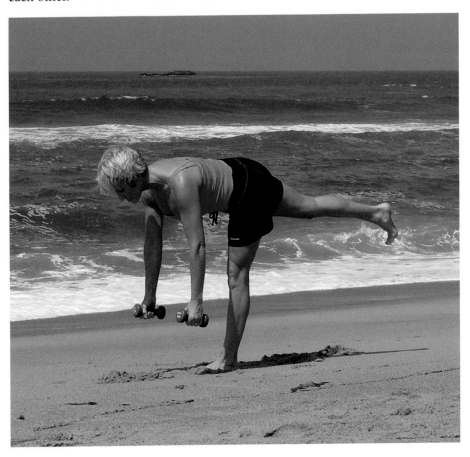

Inhale as you bend your elbows, bringing the weights toward your rib cage.

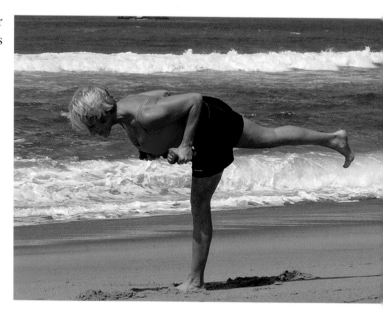

Exhale as you extend the weights toward your hips. Bend the elbows and return your arms to the starting position. Repeat 5 times before switching legs.

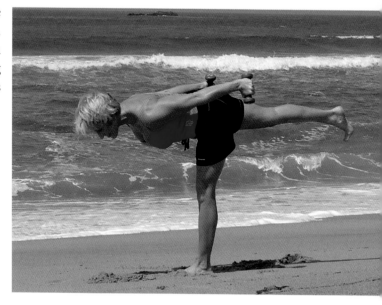

4. Side Plank (Core Balance)

Press into side plank as shown. Hold for 3–5 breaths. This pose strengthens the obliques (abdominal muscles on the sides of your body).

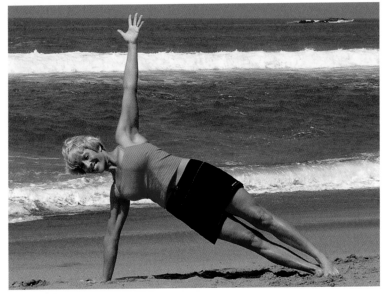

Option: Lift your top leg and hold for 3 breaths. Repeat sequence on the other side.

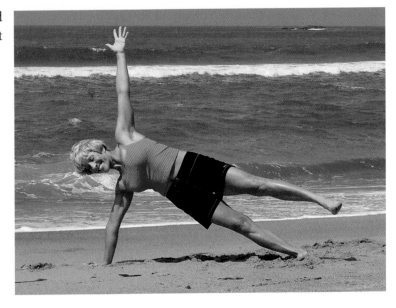

5. Standing Pigeon (Stretch)

Cross one ankle over your thigh and bend both knees. Stretch your torso be extending your arms overhead. Hold for 5 breaths and switch sides.

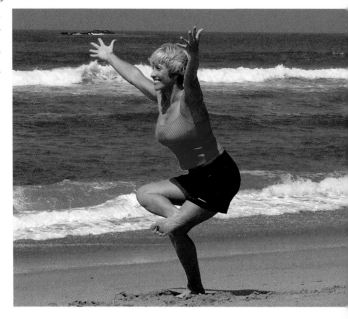

6. Standing Twist (Stretch)

This pose stretches your shoulders, chest, and spine. Lift one leg, bend the knee, and twist the torso toward the bent knee. Place the opposite hand on the outside of the raised thigh and extend the opposite arm while twisting the bent leg toward the opposite side of the body. Hold for 3–5 breaths and repeat on the other side.

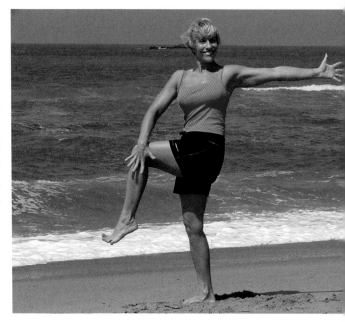

FalconGuides Interview: Get to Know Peggy Hall

Q. Who or what brought you into yoga to begin with? How did you get started and what got you hooked?

A. I was one of those people who would roll their eyes when someone mentioned yoga.

That's because I didn't think yoga could offer me anything in the way of a vigorous physical workout. To me, any activity that could provide physical benefits had to be rigorous. I had grown up as a competitive swimmer in Southern California and spent hours in the pool training. That was a workout, in my book. Later I participated in long-distance ocean swimming—very demanding and very rewarding.

As it turned out, all those years in the water took a toll on my shoulder, resulting in severe shoulder tendinitis. And my shoulder only got worse once I started surfing as an adult. In fact, I was scheduled to have shoulder surgery to alleviate my chronic pain.

Luckily, right around that time I met the man whom I would marry. And this man, David, an avid surfer himself, practiced yoga to get rid of back pain and stay fit for surfing.

This was back in the late 1990s, when yoga was just starting to get more popular. I thought yoga was only about standing on your head, burning incense, and chanting. I thought yoga was a fad that would fade away.

Was I ever wrong. I went with David to a yoga class at the community center—and that class changed my life. I never did have shoulder surgery. And my surfing improved dramatically.

I started looking around for a surf-specific yoga series—but nothing existed! I knew that yoga and surfing were a natural fit—both yoga and surfing are about being alive in each moment, aware, awake, grateful for each breath, for each moment, an opportunity to go beyond time and become one with creation itself. And I knew I wanted to share my passion of yoga and surfing with the rest of the world!

So I became certified as a yoga teacher and created "Yoga for Surfers®," the first-ever surf-specific instructional DVD series—which has reached more than a quarter million surfers worldwide.

Q. What about surfing? How did that happen? Who, what, when, where, and why did you start and what has that journey been like?

A. Growing up on the beaches of Southern California, I felt at home in the water, but I secretly envied all the surfers riding waves.

Back in the 1980s, not many females were in the lineup at that time . . . and this was before the days of female surf camps—in fact, before the days of surf lessons in general! It seemed like surfing was off-limits for all but the most die-hard female surfers.

Fortunately, times began to change, and on a trip to Kauai (back in the late 1990s) I decided to take the plunge and signed up for surf lessons.

I remember trying to stand up on that ten-foot foam board, and I was so frustrated because I could not find my balance! I was certain that my background as an ocean swimmer would make surfing a breeze, so why was I struggling? I could not believe how challenging it was to get to my feet and then to steer the board in the direction I wanted it to go.

All those surfers of my childhood memories glided so effortlessly, so magically, so euphorically on those sparkling swells—so why couldn't I do the same? That is precisely what got me hooked: my determination to master the art of riding waves with effortless ease and pure stoke!

When I got back to California, divine intervention directed me to the man who would become my husband. David was a lifelong surfer and thrilled that I wanted to get into surfing. It was a match made in heavenly swells.

David put me on a regular shortboard, which was much easier for me to handle. He took me right out into the lineup—no learning in the soup for me—and my destiny was sealed. Me, David, and a lifetime of waves.

I feel most at home when I'm in the water. There are not many things I would rather do than surf, as it makes me feel refreshed, exhilarated, alive! I may not be the best or most experienced surfer out there, but I consider myself one of the most passionate surf-stoked yogis around.

I like to say that it's not about the wave count; it's about making each wave count. And . . . sometimes the wipeout *is* the ride.

Being in the ocean, experiencing the totality of what it is to be a surfer: getting to the beach, sussing the conditions, warming up before paddling out, taking note of the weather, the ocean conditions, the lineup, and the tides, feeling the temperature of the water, smelling and tasting the salt air, breathing in the goodness of life itself—surfing is a transcendent activity that grabs the heart and soul and never lets go.

Q. Can you describe your first or most transcendent experience with yoga? Anything that made you experience the flow state we are talking about in this book?

A. Not long after I started practicing yoga, my body went through a healing crisis—unlike anything I've ever experienced before or since. Likely my body was eliminating long-stored stress, pain, wounds, and emotions that needed to be released. The result was that I had an opportunity to experience yoga at its most basic and most profound element: the breath.

At one point I was so ill that I could not get out of bed. The only thing I could do was breathe. And breathe I did . . . consciously, slowly, focusing on just making it to the next breath. Inhaling life, exhaling pain.

As I focused on my breath, I realized that at its simplest, yoga was the breath. Breathing in light and energy, life itself, letting it flood and feed my body with healing cleansing energy, and then exhaling out pain and discomfort and letting myself feel calm and connected.

Each breath, a prayer of gratitude. Each breath, a gift of life.

Q. What about surfing? Was there an experience that stands out more than the rest, and can you describe it in words? Where were you?

A. For me, every day surfing is a new glorious adventure! I can look back on some amazing waves and certain spectacular sessions when I felt transported into a magical moment that transcended time . . . completely at one with the ocean, at one with creation. Elation is what I call it.

One day in particular, we were getting footage for the *Yoga for Surfers* videos in Carlsbad, California. We were at Ponto's on a beautiful, clear, warm spring morning. A pod of dolphins showed up in the lineup, which they often do, but this time was different.

The dolphins joined us on every wave as if to say, "This is how it's done"— literally surfing with us, encouraging us to ride faster, with more joy. I shared a wave with one of these elegant, playful, giant, gray bottlenose acrobats, and when I turned to paddle back out, this same dolphin leapt right in front of me, launching several feet into the air, splashing down with exuberance, and then flip, flip, flipped his way back out to the lineup.

I remember thinking that even if I died that moment, my life would be complete.

Q. Are there specific places on earth (I call these energy vortexes) where you feel most connected to this energy or flow state of consciousness, whether you are practicing yoga, surfing, both, or just being?
A. Creation is so magnificent, so vast and so varied—such a beautiful metaphor for the soul.

I feel at home in the ocean and equally moved by vast desert spaces. Desert sand dunes remind me of ocean waves, captivating and endless.

However, the place on earth where I feel most connected, the place I feel is the most powerful energy vortex, is in the depths of my own soul, which has expanded to hold all of life's treasures. Whether practicing yoga, surfing, or just being, when I connect my body, brain, and breath and spend time in heartfelt gratitude, I find the place where power meets peace, and love meets life.

Q. Can you name your favorite surf break and where that is? What about for new surfers, is there a best place to learn in your opinion? Did you start with lessons or just go out and take the waves on? Is your family into surfing or were you a pioneer in your family?
A. If I could only surf one break for the rest of my life, it would be Middles (Trestles). Middles is the uncrowded sibling of Lowers, and there are plenty of peaks and waves for everybody. Trestles is part of the California State Park system, so thankfully it is protected, remote, and beautiful.

The beauty of the Trestles surf experience starts with a journey—on a bike, a skateboard, or on foot. The remoteness of Trestles invites you to leave your daily life behind and draw closer to raw creation. I find that as I hike toward the surf break, my mind clears, my heart opens, and my breath deepens. Stress of the day dissolves into the simplicity of sea, sand, and surf, and all is right with the world.

For new surfers, my advice is to start out at a surf spot that is safe and forgiving. Obtain local knowledge by talking to lifeguards or other surfers. Surf with a buddy. Consider taking surf lessons.

New and experienced surfers alike can benefit from my *Ocean Confidence Handbook* (available at yogaforsurfers.com), full of handy tips that help surfers get the most out of this thrilling experience! Even experienced surfers can benefit from learning more about how to know the ocean better, how to read the waves, and how to stay safe in order to catch more waves, surf them better than ever, and have more fun while doing so.

When I first started learning how to surf as an adult, my husband (whom I was dating at the time) got me up and riding on the waves right out in the lineup! He figured that since I was at home in the water as an ocean swimmer, it suited my nature to get right out there on a shortboard and take my lumps. I used to get so frustrated with myself, and often my surf session ended with me in tears on the beach.

That was before I discovered yoga.

I reluctantly tried yoga (I originally thought yoga was just for hippies) to help heal my severe shoulder tendinitis; not only did my shoulder heal, but my surfing also improved dramatically. I felt stronger, more flexible, more fit and conditioned, and my mental outlook was more calm and centered, too. Wiping out or missing waves didn't bother me as much as it used to—and I was catching more waves than ever.

I was so passionate about my yoga and surfing connection that I became certified as a yoga instructor and then set about sharing my passion with tens of thousands of surfers around the world with my *Yoga for Surfers* videos.

Yoga helps you stay calm and focused in challenging situations so you remain aware, alive, and centered in your own essence, staying balanced, calm, open, and free. You learn to connect to that deepest part of yourself so your surfing can be the unique expression of your own power, energy, and spirit.

(See also my answer to question 2.)

Q. Where and how did you start out in yoga? What was your first introduction to the practice and how do you suggest people start if they are considering getting into yoga? What is your favorite style to practice? Do you teach yoga? If so, what style?

A. For those starting out in yoga, keep in mind that yoga is as vast as art, music, or food. Keep trying different classes, teachers, and styles until you find a class, teacher, and style that suits you.

Even if you've tried yoga before and it wasn't a good fit for you, give it a try again. Yoga is a powerful practice that will benefit your physical health, emotional outlook, and mental fitness and can cross over into all areas of your life, bringing a greater sense of well-being, calm, and peacefulness.

I developed and teach my own style of surf-specific yoga called Yoga for Surfers (yogaforsurfers.com), which I pioneered back in 2002. Yoga for Surfers is a fun, fluid, and flowing style of feel-good yoga that focuses on stretching and strengthening all the muscles used in surfing, with an emphasis on the neck and shoulders, core, back, and hips. Tens of thousands of surfers around the world have used the *Yoga for Surfers* instructional videos to get fit, focused, and fearless on the waves—and on the waves of life!

(See also my answer to question 1 about how I got started in yoga.)

Q. Do you feel a beginner can access the feeling of the flow state either in yoga or surfing or would you say it's more of an advanced practice that they can work their way up to with consistent dedicated practice?

A. When you connect the mind and body with the energy of the breath, amazing things happen! Whether you're new to yoga or surfing, or a passionate practitioner, the beauty of both yoga and surfing is that the pure stoke is available to everyone.

The key to finding your flow—whether in surfing or yoga—is to breathe, relax, focus on the positive, and enjoy, enjoy, enjoy. Each breath is a gift, each moment a glorious adventure.

Approach each pose, each wave, each practice with cheerful curiosity and positive expectations that the best is yet to come. Encourage yourself positively, saying things like: "I got this! I'm getting it! I look forward to improving in this area!" Encouraging yourself will dramatically accelerate your enjoyment in both surfing and yoga.

Be patient if you feel you're backsliding. That is a part of life. Keep your head above the waves and find the peace within.

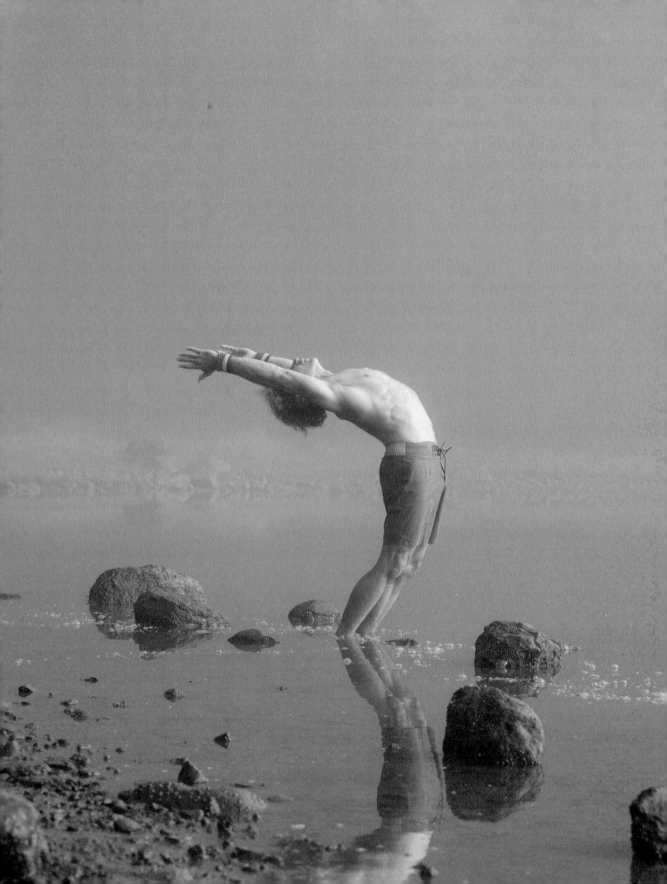

BLISSOLOGY
Eoin Finn

This morning I woke up and told the ocean I was sorry.
I kept myself in a box
I lived inside the four walls of my own problems
But when I stood beside the ocean, a warm wind
entered my heart
I realized that the beauty I see lives in me
This morning I woke up and told the ocean I was sorry
that I forgot that I am this infinity.

—*Eoin Finn*

About Eoin

Life-changing, mystical, shamanistic, radical, and hilariously funny are only a few of the adjectives tossed around to describe Eoin Finn by his blissful following of students from across the globe. The Canadian native is a globally renowned yogi, surfer, and Blissologist who has been carving his original tracks through the metaphysical worlds of yoga, philosophy, and movement since 1989.

Eoin has been lauded by Yoga Journal *magazine as "the Thoreau of Yoga" for his eco-activism and dedication to connecting yogis more deeply to the spirituality of nature, and by Oprah as "one to watch." His down-to-earth spirituality refreshes like cool water, and his Blissology Yoga style centers on the simple idea of sharing happiness. He believes that to find bliss you must "seek quiet solitude in nature and your deepest heart will be known."*

In 1999 Eoin founded a yoga system called Blissology exploring strategies for bringing more joy, awe, love, and bliss into our lives. Blissology is about mining for the source of love inside all of us that is especially evident when we are quiet and present in nature.

A Blissology Yoga class strikes the perfect balance between our ego drive and the infinitely kind and wise side of ourselves so that we treat our bodies, our communities, and nature more sustainably and with more reverence. He has a gift for making complex concepts easy to grasp and exudes enthusiasm in his teachings. In particular he is passionate about bringing spirituality down to earth and reclaiming quiet time in nature as the greatest spiritual portal and our best source of health and happiness.

His visionary writings about health, happiness, and interconnection have appeared alongside noted authors Deepak Chopra, Prince Charles, and Eckhart Tolle, and include features in Vogue, InStyle, Yoga Journal, *and* Oprah Magazine.

Fusing his passion for athletics and yoga, Eoin has prepared over one hundred Olympians as well as pro athletes from around the world for high-level competition.

Eoin's teachings offer a heart-opening, invigorating, and experiential practice, grounded with humor, dynamism, and a focus on both physical and energetic alignment, not to mention some great yoga grooves inspired by his love for surfing and the ocean. Yoga, when practiced with this holistic awareness, becomes fluid therapy, movement guided by the innate knowledge of our anatomy and evolution.

A passionate ocean activist, Eoin started the Blissology EcoKarma project in 2014, raising aid and awareness through yoga and activism for the world's precious but imperiled coral reefs. Thus far, he has helped replant over one square kilometer of coral reef in the Florida Keys and continues this work in Australia, North America, and Indonesia today.

He counts among his teachers Ravi Ravindra, Nadia Toraman, David Swenson, David Williams, Pattabhi Jois, Nancy Gilgoff, Donna Holleman, Orit Sen Gupta, Gioia Irwin, myofascial alignment teacher Tom Myers, and body-mind psychotherapist Susan Aposhyan and Bonnie Bainbridge Cohen of Body-Mind Centering. He also studied karate in Osaka, Japan, for many years, a discipline that is infused into the holistic body-mind-heart experience of Blissology Yoga.

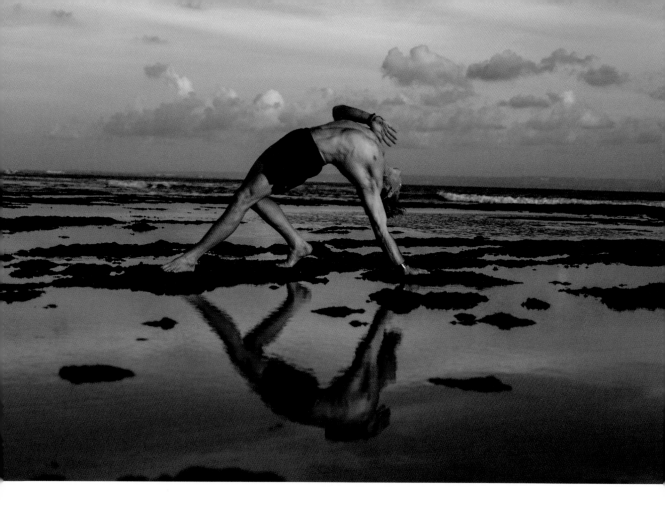

Eoin's Tips for Yoga and Surfing Success

Do it for the joy. In both yoga and surfing, we have a tendency to want to prove we are as good as someone next to us. This ruins the state of flow and turns what we love into another rat race. Of course we still want to make progress, but this will be a by-product of making our yoga and surfing a joyous expression of being alive.

Blur the line where you end and where nature begins. Feel the wind in your breath, feel the ocean in your veins, and the bright sun in the center of your chest. Each wave is a gift from the other side of the world that will never come again. In a yoga pose or surfing a wave, we are riding a miracle.

Relax into the present. There is nowhere else to be than right here and now. The amount of joy we get from surfing and yoga is directly proportionate to how in the moment we are. This means our body and mind are only responding to what is happening in this moment and are not caught up in the past or tight because we are thinking about the future. Tension in the body serves no practical purpose. It ruins the fluidity of our movements. But most importantly, when we are tight, we are trying to be someone else. When we are relaxed, we are our own true nature: the bliss of each unfolding moment.

This is the secret of yoga, surfing—and life.

FalconGuides Interview: Get to Know Eoin Finn

Q. Who or what brought you into yoga to begin with? How did you get started and what got you hooked?

A. One of the main questions I have been continuously exploring since I was a young boy is, "What happens mentally, physiologically, and spiritually when we seek quiet solitude in the beauty of nature?"

Ever since I was young, I felt a profound connection to all life in nature. I believe that all life is a miracle, that we are all intimately connected, that we share the same source, and that there is a deep peace at the core of our being. In daily life, unfortunately, stress, tension, and worry cover this place up. When we are in nature, the lines between where we end and nature begins disappear.

When I was a teenager, I became very interested in the teachings of Joseph Campbell. He talked about the idea of Brahman as the ultimate energy source. It is not a white-bearded man in the sky who judges us for right and wrong, but it is pure transcendent energy. It transcends the mind. It is not God the concept but God the experience. This is what I felt in nature. I was fascinated, and it led me to study Eastern philosophy and yoga in university.

I learned meditation and pranayama first, then added a few basic yoga routines that I practiced on my own in the morning overlooking the Mediterranean Sea in France where I finished my schooling. It was magical, but I didn't know the proper alignment or the gymnastic elements.

This I learned when I moved to Maui in 1995. I dropped into a yoga class led by Nadia Toraman. It was Ashtanga based, and it was so hard I almost died. I had never thought of yoga as exercise. I thought its purpose was to restore balance after vigorous exercise. Even though I was tight and stiff from all of my other sports, I knew I would do it until the day I died. Yoga was like the temple, the university, and the gym all wrapped into one.

Q. What about surfing? How did that happen? Who, what, when, where, and why did you start and what has that journey been like?

A. I learned surfing, tai chi, meditation, and yoga all in the same year. It was 1988, my second year of university.

I was a windsurfer first and spent a lot of time windsurfing at Lawrencetown Beach, not far from Halifax, Nova Scotia. I met a lot of the surf community out there and decided not to pay rent for the first three months of college but to pay "tent." I bought a tent and pitched it for three months on a beautiful point over-looking the beach. It was great for my soul, but not so good for my homework.

By December I had moved indoors due to the weather. One of my surfing friends I had met called me up at 6:00 a.m. on a January morning. "Today is going to be epic!" he told me on the phone as I rolled out of bed.

I looked out the window and told him, "It's totally dark . . . and it's snowing!" It was minus six degrees Celsius.

"No problem, I have a 5mm wetsuit for you and warm gloves. You'll be fine."

He was right. If you are hardy enough to brave the weather, Nova Scotia has an endless supply of legendary point breaks. He loaned me a seven-foot Mini Mal surfboard, and I walked through the snow to get to the break.

The water was so glassy, and the cold stinging on my face had turned to stoke. After eating it several times on the takeoff, around my third attempt I paddled in and went down the line about one hundred yards.

It was like becoming a dolphin or an eagle. It was happiness distilled. I was in flow. There was nowhere else to be. My body knew supreme joy, and from that point on there was no turning back. My friends were hollering and the barrier between nature and my soul disappeared. I knew that I would never see the world the same again and that my life would be dedicated to re-creating the pure joy of that first glide.

You never forget your first wave.

Q. Can you describe your first or most transcendent experience with yoga? Anything that made you experience the flow state we are talking about in this book?

A. It's hard to pinpoint one transcendent experience in yoga that stands out above the rest. Instead it is a stream of thousands of transcendental moments on the mat. To say which one is more powerful than another is as hard as naming your favorite child.

What has changed for me over the years is the idea of transcending. When I studied transcendental meditation, I used to think that I would transcend material reality and enter the spiritual realm. It was a release from the world of concepts and forms. I thought I would go to another dimension.

What I've realized on my path, though, is that instead of transcending reality, I go deeper into the very fibers of it. It isn't a transcendent escape from reality but a deep dive into its very essence.

What I transcend is my self-limiting thoughts about who I am. I am no longer limited by concepts of a lower vibration: what's going wrong in my life, what I need to get done, or how I wish something had never happened to me.

I transcend those thoughts and enter a realm of my highest vibrational self: Time is less crushing, life is a miracle, there is a feeling of light expanding from my heart that reminds me I am intimately connected to all life, from the fish in the oceans to people on the other side of the planet. I am reminded that we all have a calling to bring more love and joy into the world. No longer am I in resistance to the way things are but in flow with it.

I know when this happens best in my practice. At the very end, after savasana (the relaxation part), every Blissology Yoga practice ends with what we call a "Circle of Light." Something biologically happens when we gather close to other people in a circle that doesn't happen as easily when we sit on our mats in our private little rectangles. Our ancestors knew this, and that's why so many of the world's great traditions met in circles. When we are closer to people around us, we feel the essence of their hearts more. Our inner mammal finds pleasure in this and so does our inner angel.

When pushed to describe the best moment like this, I would say it was at Wanderlust Oahu in 2015. I taught a class there and Nahko played music for it. At the end of the yoga practice, three hundred or so bodies all huddled around each other in a Circle of Light in a carpeted ballroom at the Turtle Bay Resort. We relaxed into our breath, establishing a flow state by making it long, slow, and deep. Wherever there is excessive tension tells a story. There is fear or a wound there that needs to move out.

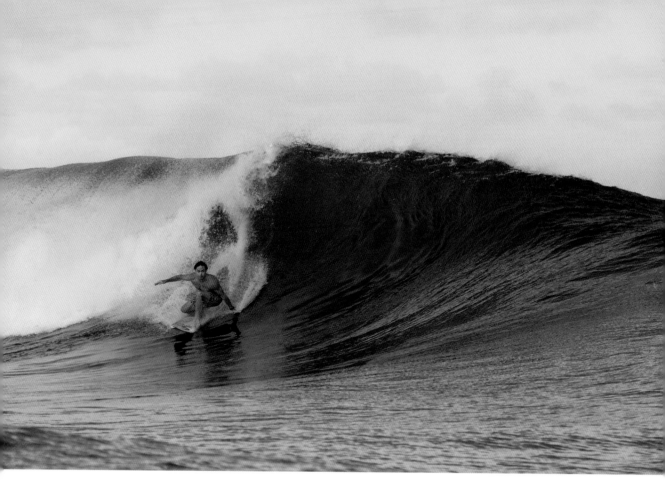

Q. What about surfing? Was there an experience that stands out more than the rest, and can you describe it in words? Where were you?

A. It's always surfing with animals. Orcas, fish, whales, but I remember one encounter in particular with a sea lion I named Salmie that I will never forget.

It's a warm autumn day on Wickaninnish Beach on the west coast of Vancouver Island. I've surfed all over the world, and it is getting harder and harder to find places to surf that aren't covered in condos, hotels, or restaurants. I leave the parking lot with my new red surfboard under my arm. I pass the coolness of the forest that never leaves this part of the world even on sunny days, bare feet hitting warm sand as I run past piles of driftwood stretching for miles along the coastline—gray and faded, weather-worn temples to the power of elements here: the wind, the sea, and the endless rain.

There is a deep joy animating everyone on the beach today that normally only those with four legs can feel. I tune in to it, feeling like a child running to the beach. I watch my friend catch a wave, slashing, water spraying, and I can't wait for my turn.

Every time I enter the ocean, the very instant my head goes under the water I understand why it has always been used to cleanse the soul—from John the Baptist to a Brahman in the Ganges River. Any worry or preoccupation I have ever felt washes off me, and I am living what I try and teach people all the time: deep presence. I feel the cool water surrounding me, but I am warm in my wetsuit.

I search out the most likely place for a rideable wave to break, following a trail of sea foam. I know this is where the biggest sets will unload.

It's my turn. I am like a dog with a bone, practically growling with a big dose of wahoo as I launch into a steep wall of water that has traveled thousands of miles from Japan to its explosive ends here on this remote beach.

I see a shadowy figure as I take the last stroke and jump to my feet. In a millisecond my brain makes the computation: Shark? No, too small. Sea lion . . . I am on this wave with a damn sea lion! As I ride the wave, he bumps my board continuously. It's more than a little disconcerting. What does he want? Am I a competitor in his fishing zone?

The wave ends and I am off my board in the water; I can see the light beige fur as he bumps me. I am in the food chain now. His body feels fishy and slick, but simultaneously furry and muscled like a horse. Not many people get to feel this, but frankly I'd rather not.

I am not romanticizing this situation. I still can't tell if he is being playful or aggressive. I try and project telepathically to him that I am not here for his women; I'm married and just passing through.

I get back on my board, feeling slightly safer than when my limbs were dangling in the water. More bumps from this sea lion. He's going crazy. Swimming under me, around me. It's like a very uncomfortable game of whack-a-mole. Where will he pop up next?

I catch wave after wave, and it's the same scenario. I just can't shake this guy, and the jury is still out on whether he is an overly enthusiastic friend or foe. I start to think of him more as the former, but even if he is friendly, one overly playful nip from him means "goodbye, little finger for me."

My friends are laughing at me, and I shrug as I paddle in to the beach. I walk about 400 yards up the beach and relaunch my board. Thank God that's over.

But it's not. I haven't even made it to the lineup yet and he is back. Bumping me and getting in the way of every wave I ride. I feel that "fish fur" on my skin one too many times and head in to the beach. My session is over, and I go home a little upset that I didn't even get one good wave in before that frisky light beige sea lion ruined my session.

The next day I arrive at the beach, and it's back to a more typical West Coast drizzle. The waves are smaller, and I see a small pack of surfers way down the beach.

I paddle out, enjoying the silence. You can hear every drop of water landing in the ocean and the swish of my hands paddling through glass-calm water.

I wait for the sets to arrive, and suddenly the beige fur, large whiskers, and huge eyes pop up out of the water. I am more trusting of his intentions today since nothing bad happened yesterday. He is less jumpy, and we wait patiently for the waves to arrive.

Finally a shoulder-high wave breaks and I paddle into it. I see the shadow of the sea lion in the wave in front of me. The wave is propelling him, and he looks like a large eagle soaring on the breeze in front of me. I do turns over the top of him, amazed at our synchronicity.

The wave ends and I am off my board again, but no slimy, furry body hits me. It's a much more tranquil affair. As I paddle back out, those whiskers and curious eyes are right beside me, and I can't help but think of the first human that befriended a wolf and created dogs.

We wait for another wave. He's simply looking at me; I'm looking at him.

"What's your name?" I casually ask. "Hmmm . . . how about Salmie, like Salmon? Let's call you Salmie the Sea Lion!"

Another wave comes, another incredible dance with this surprisingly graceful creature under my board. We paddle back out again and again.

There was a time in my life when I would go to zoos not so much to see the animals but to photograph children looking at animals. What is that connection? Arms would always be outstretched, jaws open. It was a universal look. Why do we light up around animals like this? What primordial bond do we share?

When I was young, my grandmother always asked me what I wanted to be when I grew up. "An Indian!" I always replied, to her dismay. Not a fireman or a doctor. I wanted a life where I could walk shoulder to shoulder with brother wolf and sister moon.

Next month I will be in Bombay, India, in a land I have married. This is the birthplace of yoga. It occurred to me on my last trip that there are millions of people on this planet who will never walk barefoot on the grass or on the beach. Not just people in the slums but the middle class with their feet jammed in dress shoes even at luxury resorts on the coast. It makes me think about all the times I have taught yoga in conference centers that are two levels below street level on carpet with no view, teaching people about health and spirituality.

Spirituality to me *is* nature. Religions try and answer the question of what happens when we die? Do we have a soul? Who created this whole show we call life? Who is in charge? I think about these questions continuously and I can't answer them still. Can anyone?

I don't feel a need to anymore. The imperative of our generation is to bring spirituality down to earth, not up to heaven.

I am clear that my path is not about what happens when we die, but about the joy we feel knowing that the same salt that makes up our oceans runs through our veins. In yoga class, I encourage people to taste their salty sweat lest they think that happiness comes from asana alone. Every tear, every drop of sweat comes and goes from the ocean. Our cells wouldn't divide if we hadn't learned to trap salt water inside of us.

Mother Theresa said, "The problem with humans is we forget that we belong to each other," and she's right. That's only half the problem, though; we also forget we belong to nature.

When I die, if I can help to keep future generations focused on what I feel is the greatest source of happiness—our mystical interconnection to all life—I will consider this the best afterlife of all. During this lifetime, I just want to keep my heart ignited by this beauty.

People ask me all the time who my greatest teachers were. This list is long, and I am so grateful to stand on the shoulders of giants. All I have to transmit ultimately is the energy that lights up my soul from the beauty of interconnection.

I am still paddling out through the surf. I duck under a wave. The cold water cleanses my thoughts. Baptizing me deeper into a perspective where I can feel the ocean around me and inside me. I taste the salt in the water. This salt is my blood. It's the blood of Salmie. I howl inside with happiness!

Q. Are there specific places on earth where you feel most connected to this energy or flow state of consciousness, whether you are practicing yoga, surfing, both, or just being?
A. Anywhere we haven't paved is superpowerful and opens us up to the energy of life and nature, what the Hawaiians call mana. I would say one place I feel this the most is in W.A. (Western Australia). The beaches around Margret River blow me

away. There is just so much raw power there. The surf is punchy, often on rocky slabs, and there are miles and miles of empty beaches as far as the eye can see. I love it all—the color of the light sand, the vastness of the sky, the turquoise water in the shallows turning deep blue. Even the sharks remind me of this power. Not far inland there is an abundance of food in this Mediterranean climate: vineyards, olive plantations, and so many farmers' markets. I feel the ruggedness of my own heart when I am there. I feel it in the people.

There are a lot of places I feel this: Santa Cruz, Raglan, New Zealand, and up in British Columbia. Of course, there is also nothing like the mana of Hanalei Bay, Kauai, to plug my life force into a vortex of the earth's energy.

Let's hope these places never get paved, mined, or turned into golf courses. Raw beauty is a portal to the soul.

Q. Can you name your favorite surf break and where that is? What about for new surfers, is there a best place to learn in your opinion? Did you start with lessons or just go out and take the waves on? Is your family into surfing or were you a pioneer in your family?

A. From a pure surfing perspective, I love the Mentawai Islands of Indonesia. I love the power of the ocean out there and how removed I am from technology. I put away my smartphone and open up my "heart phone" the whole time I am there. My eyes never leave the ocean, whether I am on the surf paddling until my arms fall off or sitting in a hammock watching the surf from a distance. I am under its spell.

I never started with formal lessons, although I always advise beginners to do this, telling them how surfing is the hardest sport in the world. Just knowing where to sit to catch a wave has a long learning curve. I got pummeled learning—breaking boards, getting pitched over the falls, being held under the water.

Somehow this is such a great analogy for life. When we are clear about what our passions are, life is going to initiate us. It will ask us, "How badly do you want this?" Are you willing to work for it and get drilled to the bottom or do you want to just quit and go sit on a lounge chair like all those people you see back on the beach?

I learned this teaching yoga. When I first started, nobody showed up to my classes. It was me and an empty room. My spirit was dejected. I knew this was what I was meant to do, but the universe initiated me when I wanted to follow my dreams the same way it initiated me when I learned to surf.

I tell this story to all the people who do our teacher trainings. Joseph Campbell said, "Follow your bliss and doors will open where once there were walls." What I have realized he never mentioned is that these doors will open when the universe makes us go deep inside ourselves and answer the question: "How badly do you want this?"

For both surfing and teaching yoga, I'm so glad I answered this call.

Q. Where and how did you start out in yoga? What was your first introduction to the practice and how do you suggest people start if they are considering getting into yoga? What is your favorite style to practice? Do you teach yoga? If so, what style?

A. My first experiences with yoga asana came after I had studied meditation and yoga philosophy. I wanted so badly to learn the poses, but I had no teacher. I bought a book and tried to learn. I was super stiff and it wasn't easy. During one summer, I had a friend whose mom was a yoga teacher. If you want to do yoga, you need to learn the sun salutations, she told me. She showed me how, and it made such a difference. My body, mind, and breath became in sync. My nervous system let go of its grip on my muscles.

I practiced on my own for years. I finished my university studies in Nice, France, and would wake up at 5:00 a.m. every day to practice while watching the sun come up over the azure waters of the Mediterranean.

After college I moved to Maui. I didn't know it, but it was a mecca for Ashtanga yoga. I had no idea yoga could be that physically challenging or gymnastic. I went to a class taught by Nadia Toraman and came out dripping in sweat. I always thought of yoga as a sacred activity, but now I felt like I had gone to the temple, the university, and the gym at the same time. It was exactly what I was looking for in life. Even though I was super stiff and tight, I knew the vinyasa practice was for me.

Over the years, I drifted away from Ashtanga yoga and have learned from other styles as well as listened to the voice inside me that knows what I want to bring into the world. I now teach Blissology Yoga, which is about mining for the place of wisdom in our hearts. That place that wordlessly knows how precious and intricate our connections to others are. Then we bring this kindness out into our bodies, our personal relationships, our communities, and nature.

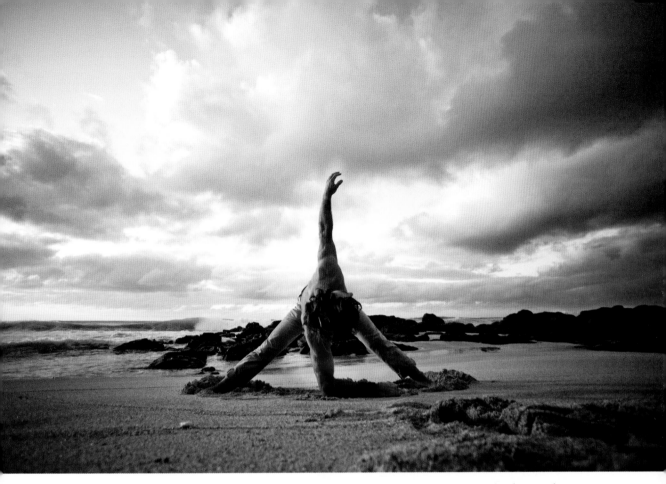

It is about becoming wiser and more sustainable to our own bodies and to the planet. It brings a therapeutic aspect to the yoga but is also about the flow of energy. It has an incredible connection to nature, and classes include time to strengthen our connection to the planet. One thing I know for sure, the more I blur the line between where I end and where nature begins, the happier I am . . . and that happiness needs to be shared!

Q. Do you feel a beginner can access the feeling of the flow state either in yoga or surfing, or would you say it's more of an advanced practice that they can work their way up to with consistent dedicated practice?
A. Yoga is the art of getting out of our own way. This happens to many people immediately after their first class. I know in my case, entering the flow state is a skill that can be better accessed by the right tools, like breath and interpreting bodily feedback. I can find the flow more easily now than I could twenty or thirty years ago. My skills have increased after years of practice.

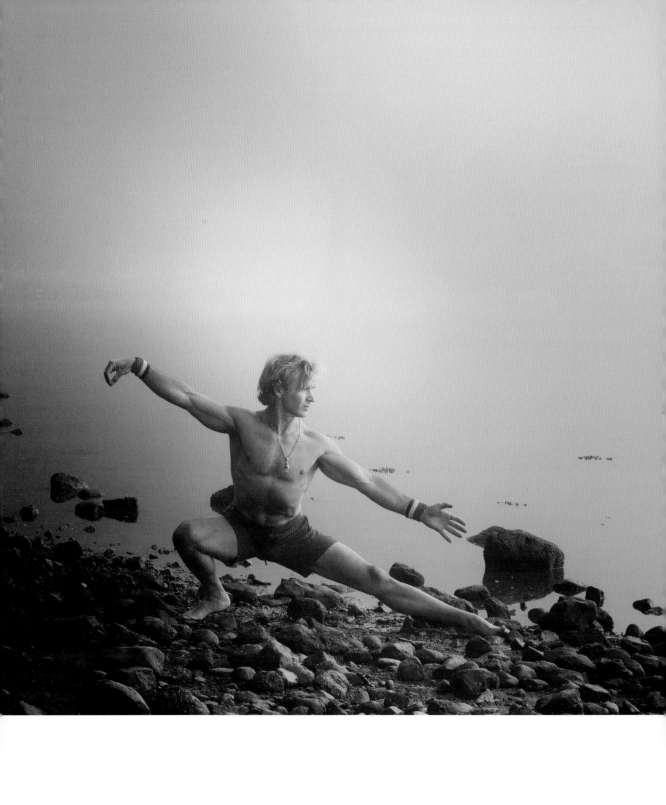

This is not to say that beginners cannot find the flow state immediately, though. It is accessible to beginners even in their first yoga class.

Flow is the absence of constriction. It happens when we are not full of self-limiting thoughts or excessive tension in our bodies. To find it, we need to remove these blocks.

In yoga, it's easy to find flow when we let go of tightness in our muscles and when our breath is relaxed and there is no secondary voice track in our head analyzing what we do, but there is just pure doing.

In surfing, these skills of knowing how to find flow pay off immediately. If we are overly tense, not connected to our breath, or have a head filled with chatter, we will probably get immediate feedback that we are not in flow with either stiff movements on the wave or a lot of wipeouts.

You probably won't fall off your yoga mat if you aren't completely in the zone, but in surfing you will. I love that it forces you to be present and in flow to do it well. I love that the elements are always moving in surfing and it isn't just our mind and body that has to be in flow like yoga, but it is a harmony of mind, body, and nature. The ocean demands our presence.

Surfing and yoga go together like the strumming and fretting hand of a guitar. They work inseparably to make a harmonious life. To me, the skills I've learned on the yoga mat have helped my surfing immeasurably. My non-surfing friends think the big benefit of yoga is flexibility, but I would say the major way yoga helps your surfing is the mental game and how much it helps us find flow.

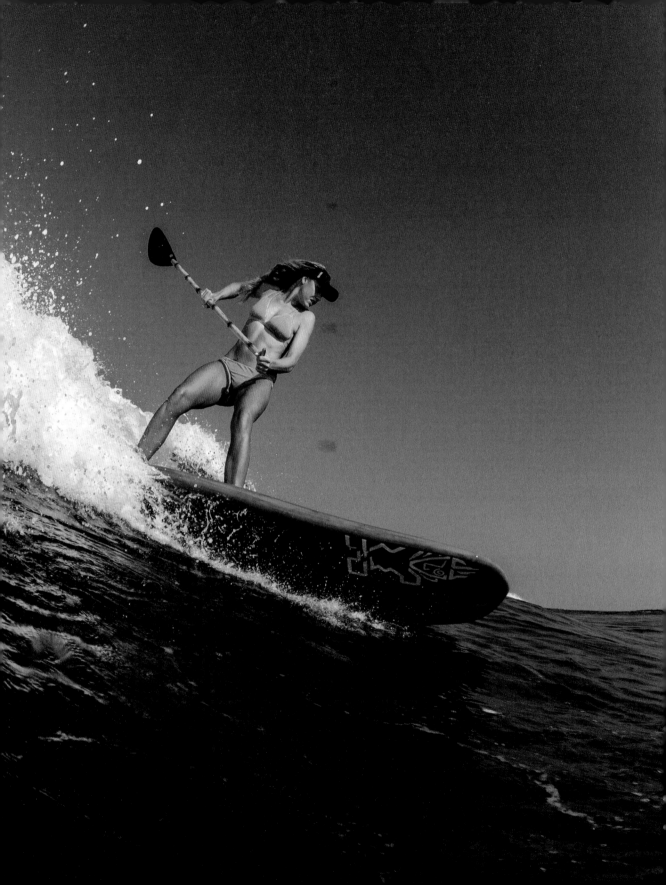

SWELL LIVING
Donica Shouse

You and I are all as much continuous with the physical universe as a wave is continuous with the ocean.

—*Alan Watts*

About Donica

Donica Shouse (Kailua Kona, Hawaii) is a multitalented water woman who excels in a wide variety of SUP disciplines. She loves SUP surfing and SUP yoga and even dabbles in downwind racing from time to time. Shouse started the first SUP yoga program on the Big Island, and she's also a huge supporter of the environment. Shouse, along with her husband, Abraham, have a media company where they film captivating underwater adventures, commercials, and weddings.

For more, visit StarShotMedia.com or follow Donica at @swellliving on both Instagram and Snapchat.

Donica's Yoga for Surfing Practice

1. Adho Mukha Svanasana or Down Dog Splits

Hold for at least 5 breaths on each side.

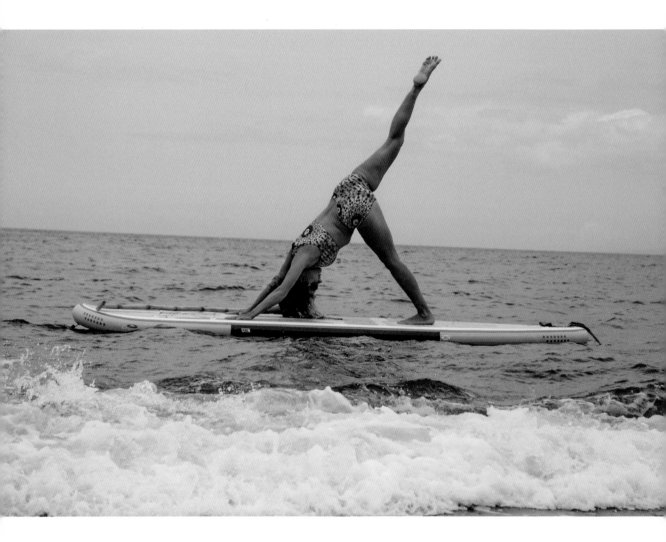

2. Eka Pada Rajakapotasana variation or Mermaid Pose

This pose requires a good deal of flexibility and is perfect for connecting to your fluid nature. Try to get in 8 full breaths here.

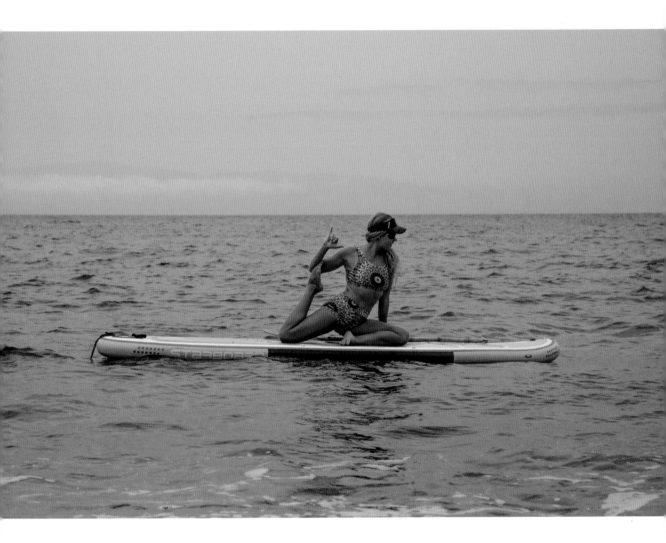

3. Parsva Balasana or Twisted Child's Pose

This pose melts my shoulders back open after a long day of surfing.

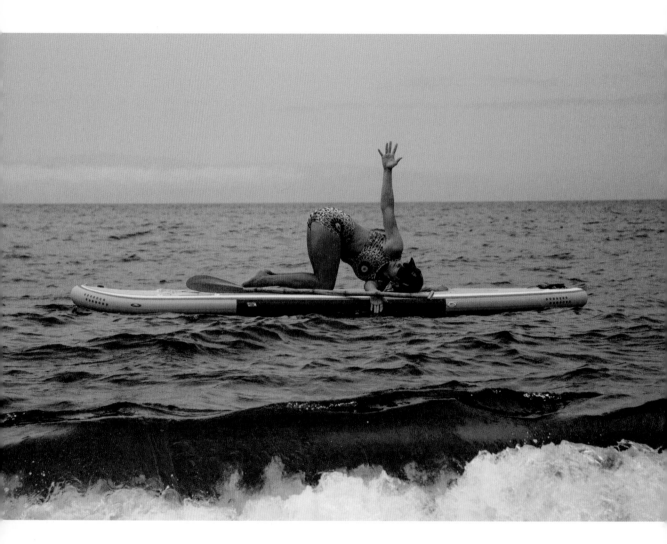

4. Ustrasana or Camel's Pose

This is a deep backbend. We bend so that we do not break.

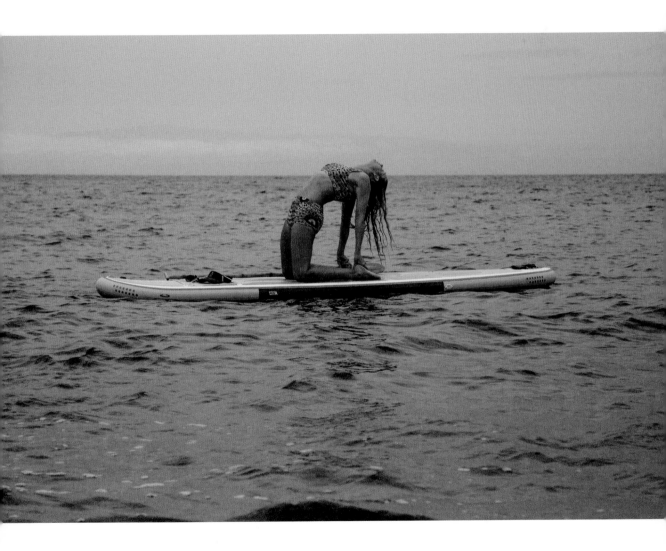

CHAPTER 5

5. Ardha Pincha Mayurasana or Dolphin Pose

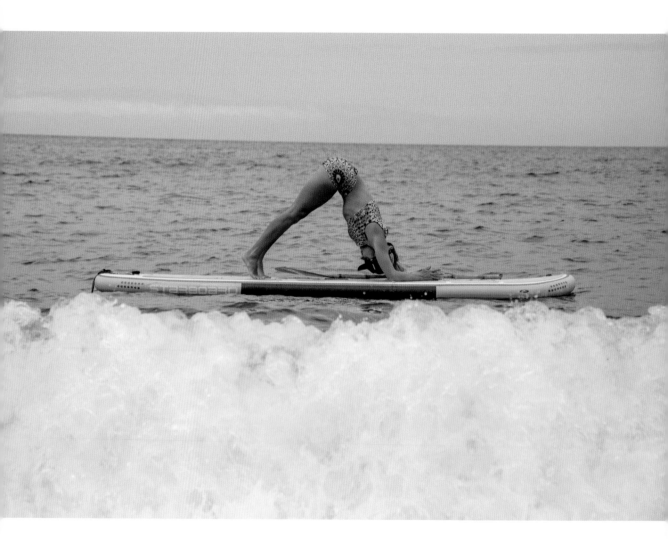

6. Salamba Sarvangasana or Shoulderstand

By turning our body upside down, we can counteract some of gravity's effects on it. Only practice this on solid ground or very calm waters.

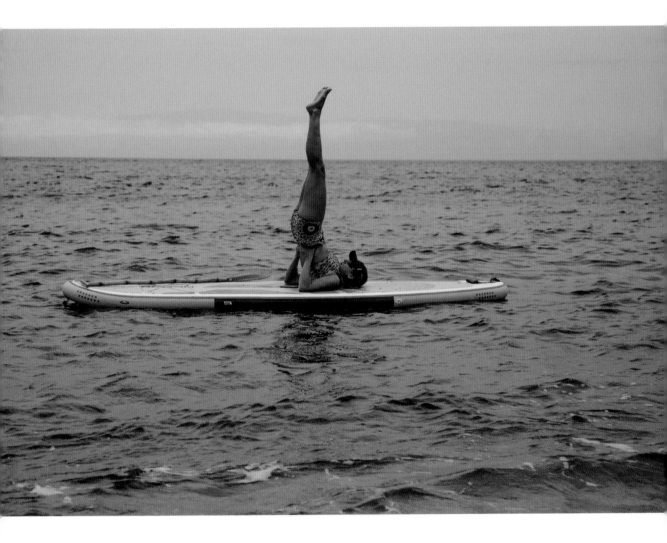

7. Mālāsana or Garland Pose

This pose is great for building strength and flexibility in the ankles. Try to stay here for 1–3 minutes.

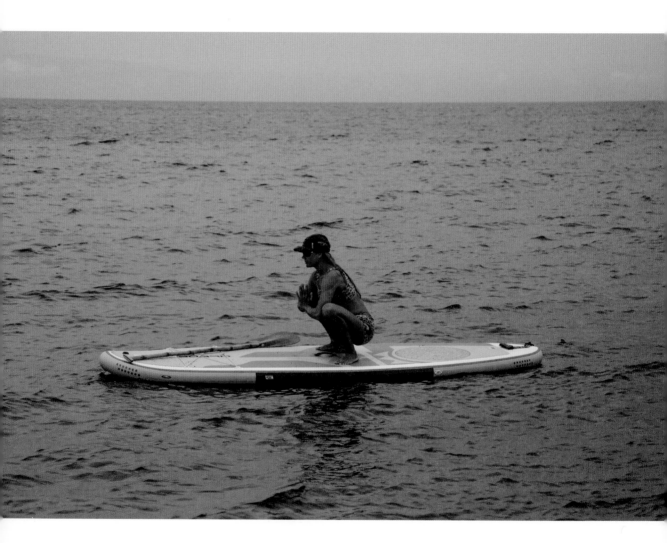

8. Bakasana or Crane Pose

This pose is great for full body engagement. Try lifting one leg at a time, building up the strength to lift both feet together. Avoid if you have a wrist or shoulder injury.

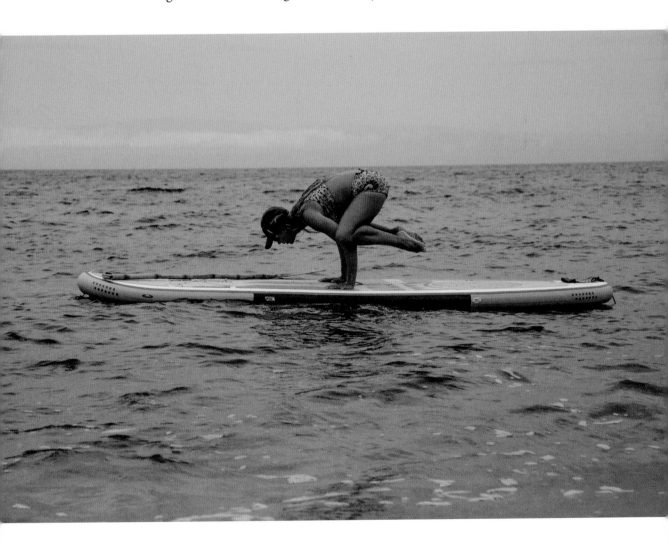

9. Balasana or Child's Pose

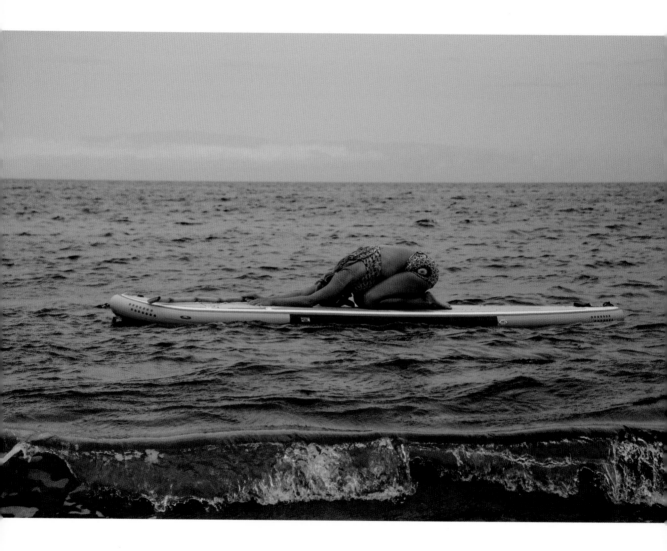

10. Bharmanasana or Balancing Table (Variation)

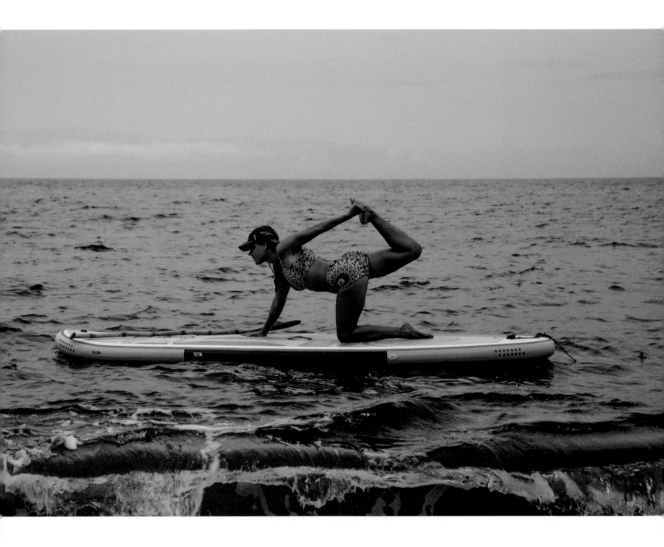

Donica's Tips for Yoga and Surfing Success

The more you eat plants, the more you want to eat plants. The bacteria in our guts have access to our thoughts and taste buds, so feed them wisely. Drink deep of freshwater first thing in the morning every day. For an added boost of energy, add matcha, maca, and spirulina to your water.

FalconGuides Interview: Get to Know Donica Shouse

Q. Who or what brought you into yoga to begin with? How did you get started and what got you hooked?

A. I got hooked on *Yoga for Surfers* from Peggy Hall. Learning to surf in Oregon is no easy feat, and I noticed immediate gains in my paddling and pop-up after pushing myself through the multiple vinyasa flows in *Yoga for Surfers* II and III. I highly recommend her post-surf yoga session, and because it's less than twenty minutes, it's pretty easy to squeeze into even the busiest of days.

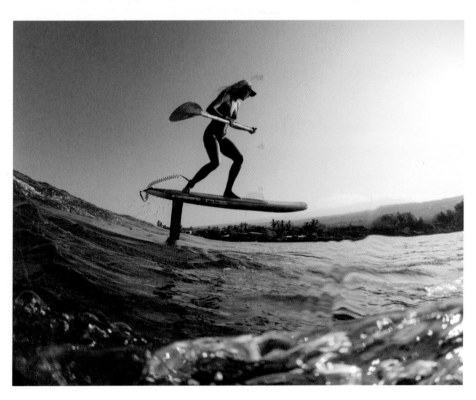

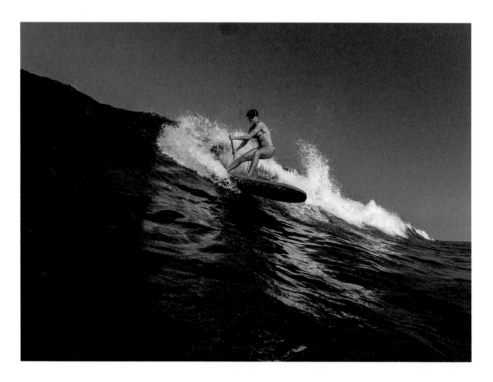

Q. What about surfing? How did that happen? Who, what, when, where, and why did you start and what has that journey been like?

A. Surf bugs are real. I caught one at age seventeen, and it's shaped my life ever since. At first, learning to surf in Oregon is also about survival—staying warm, rip currents, seaweed, logs in the surf—but I absolutely love the crispness of the waves and the curious seals. On one of my best days ever, there were icicles hanging off the headlands and frozen sheets of sand capping the beaches. After all that it was incredibly freeing to surf warm-water waves. Surfing without a wetsuit and actually feeling the board under my feet was life changing. My surf bug about doubled in size; if I could still move my arms at night, I felt like I hadn't surfed enough. So many possibilities pound our shores with each passing swell. There is not enough time in the day for all the different crafts I like to surf. I love riding alaia, shortboard, longboard, SUP, hydrofoil, canoe; even just bodysurfing can be so epic. I think it's crucial to try all the different shapes and sizes. There's always room to grow in surfing.

Q. Can you describe your first or most transcendent experience with yoga? Anything that made you experience the flow state we are talking about in this book?

A. My first yoga class left me wanting to dance and feeling tingly for about six hours. I had no idea what I was getting into. Amazing how much easier it is to move when you're properly warmed up. More recently I've fallen for hot buddha yoga, aka buti yoga, which is a fusion of dance, cardio, and yoga. I love the challenge of an asana with a thumping heartbeat and lingering desire to dance. Classes are fun, but about forty minutes of yin yoga at home puts me in the zone for the best sleeps. l like to do long-hold gravity-based stretches, so I might just do four poses in those forty minutes.

Q. What about surfing? Was there an experience that stands out more than the rest, and can you describe it in words? Where were you?

A. First time on an SUP I immediately thought how perfect for sun salutations and arm balances. Especially in Kona, so much of surfing is that meditative time between sets. SUP yoga helps me make the most of long waits between waves. Or on days when the surf is pumping nonstop, yoga post surfing helps me rejuvenate and prepare for the next day.

Q. Are there specific places on earth (I call these energy vortexes) where you feel most connected to this energy or flow state of consciousness, whether you are practicing yoga, surfing, both, or just being?

A. Such a fun question; just by the way it's phrased it points to these energy vortexes that are created in the places we spend the most time. Out of habit I always feel for that connection just before entering the ocean, and it helps me to tap into a deeper focus. Finding the flow state is just like any other practice: When you do it consistently, it becomes easier.

Q. Can you name your favorite surf break and where that is? What about for new surfers, is there a best place to learn in your opinion? Did you start with lessons or just go out and take the waves on? Is your family into surfing or were you a pioneer in your family?

A. My favorite place is in the middle of the Pacific on Hawaii's Big Island at Lyman's. It's where I met my husband surfing. Right in the heart of Kona town, this spot can handle swells of all sizes. For new surfers Kahaluu is right down the road, and I'd definitely suggest a lesson if learning on the Big Island. Compared to the other islands, Hawaii has less sand and more sharp reef, so it's a good place to hire a liaison. I learned in Oregon before there were a million tutorials on YouTube (which, by the way, are a great resource). I battled it out with a buddy in the whitewash for far too long. I probably should have gotten a lesson, but if you're persistent enough, you can pick it up bit by bit.

Q. Where and how did you start out in yoga? What was your first introduction to the practice and how do you suggest people start if they are considering getting into yoga? What is your favorite style to practice? Do you teach yoga? If so, what style?
A. I took my first yoga class in college. I enjoyed the class and really loved the lightness I felt afterward. I definitely recommend trying a variety of classes because each teacher is different. Just like every wave is different, all teachers have a unique style. As much as I enjoy the buddhi yoga, when I practice on my own I tend toward a relaxing flow to balance out my active lifestyle. And I occasionally teach private yoga-boarding classes.

Q. Do you feel a beginner can access the feeling of the flow state either in yoga or surfing, or would you say it's more of an advanced practice that they can work their way up to with consistent dedicated practice?
A. If you've experienced that flow in another sport or practice, it will transfer over. Surfing is way easier when seas are calm and likewise in yoga when the mind is calm. Success depends on the conditions you are starting with and your level of presence—yet another reason it can be helpful to have an instructor. After learning the basics, the key is repetition so muscle memory can help clear the mind.

SUP yoga boarding is such fun way to deepen your practice. After surfing I especially love side bends and twisting variations to balance out my back muscles. Dolphin is great way to extend the benefits of down dog without the added wrist strain that surfers often get enough of. Long-hold "gravity" yoga is my favorite: deep ujjayi ("ocean") breathing while holding simple stretches for three to five minutes. The ocean rocking can be very soothing during long-hold poses. Savasana at sea is something everyone should experience.

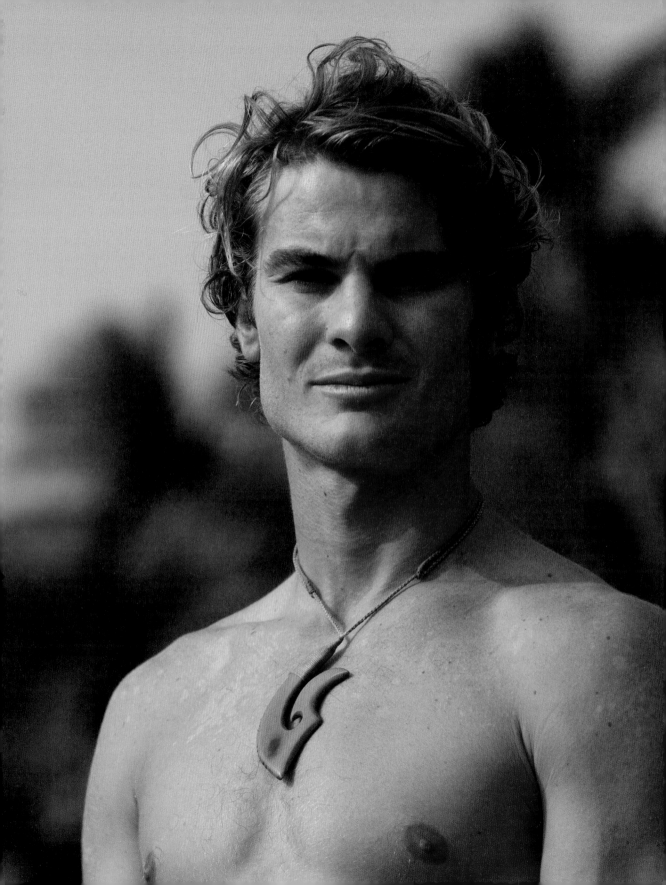

BORN TO SURF

Zane Kekoa Schweitzer

Being charismatic does not depend on how much time you have, but on how fully present you are in each interaction.

—*Olivia Fox Cabane*

About Zane

Zane has been a waterman since birth. When he's not surfing, he might be gliding through the wind kitesurfing or windsurfing, fishing with his father, diving, or training by paddling, swimming, or body-surfing. He is also an avid dirt bike racer and loves spending time flying through the mountains with his dad and brother Matty.

Zane has been fortunate enough to travel and compete around the world. At the early age of eleven years old, he was already compet-ing internationally and hasn't stopped since. He has been around the globe quite a few times and always has fun doing the multitude of sports that he loves everywhere he goes.

In 2015, Zane became 100 percent focused on achieving his dreams of being known as a waterman and world champion. He spent just as much time having fun—giving back to his community, being active in Stand Up for the Cure and hosting InZane SUPer Grom clinics—but somehow made the time to start training, really training. Zane is only now starting to scratch the surface of what he aims to conquer.

Zane finished 2015 just missing out on the title of the StandUp World Champion in SUP surfing, taking a respectable second place. But that did not satisfy him; it only fired him up and made him train even harder for 2016. He had the best year of his career, securing his third consecutive overall world championship win at the Master of the Ocean event and just weeks later taking the overall win at Red Bull's prestigious Ultimate Waterman event. Between these two events (competing in surfing, windsurfing, kitesurfing, stand-up paddle surfing, stand-up paddle racing, OC1 canoe, longboard surfing, prone paddleboarding, and swimming), Zane is now considered the best waterman in the world! His grandparents invented the sport of windsurfing, his parents were both world champions, and Zane is now the third-generation waterman pioneering his own path!

However, what Zane is most respected and loved for is the philanthropic work he does worldwide. Zane's greatest personal achievements have not been his competition results or world ranking stats; Zane cares deeply for the well-being of others and the preservation of our planet. In 2012 Zane and his family cofounded Stand Up for the Cure, a stand-up paddle event that since 2012 has raised over $650,000 for uninsured cancer patients. He founded his InZane SUPer Grom clinics, where he teaches children at home and around the world how to surf and share aloha while taking care of each other and our oceans. He is a global ambassador for multiple organizations such as Mighty Under Dogs, Access Surf, Thera Surf, Surfer's Healing, One Ocean, and more.

Recently, Zane has taken on the role of motivational speaker at schools in Hawaii and across the United States, sharing his inspirational message of "Innovate & Inspire" by sharing aloha around the world. His focus is on teaching the next generation the importance of following their dreams by finding what is important to them and then sharing it with others, as well as living a healthy and active lifestyle while taking care of the planet to make it a better place for all. Zane lives this daily.

Visit Zane's website at zaneschweitzer.com.

Zane's Yoga for Surfing Routine

1. Butterfly
Butterfly opens the inner thighs and hips.

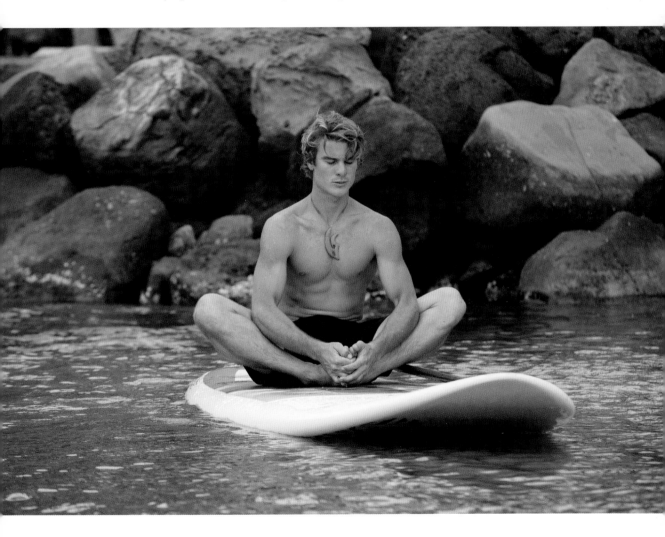

2. Butterfly with Shoulder Stretch

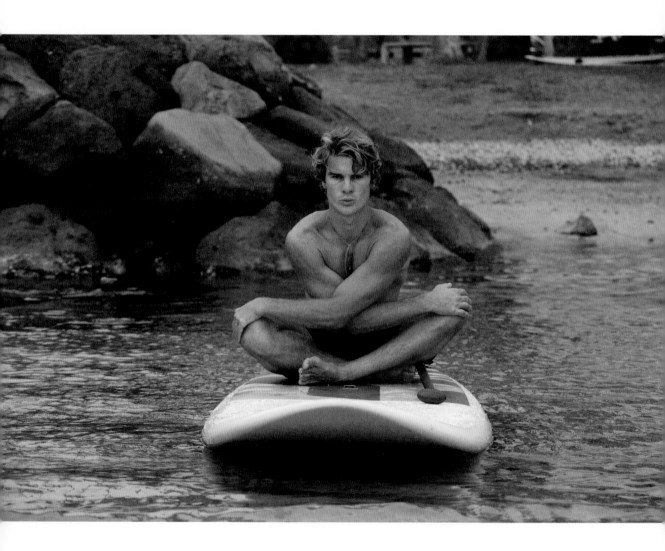

3. Downward Dog
Down dog stretches the back, hamstrings, and calves.

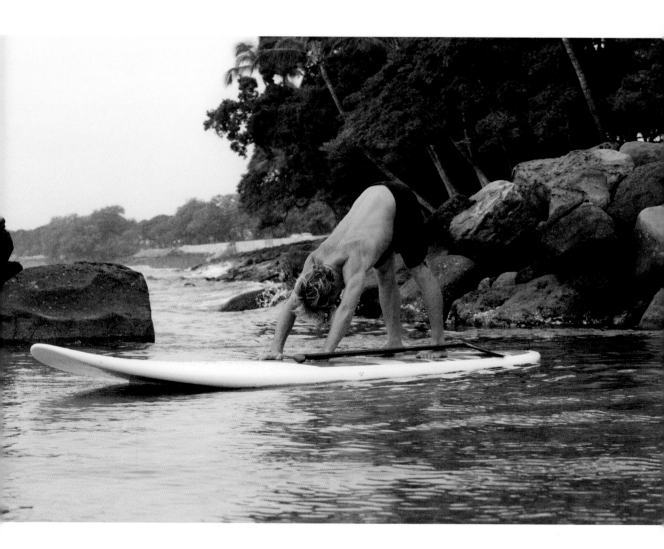

4. Upward Dog

Upward dog builds spinal flexibility and strengthens the core.

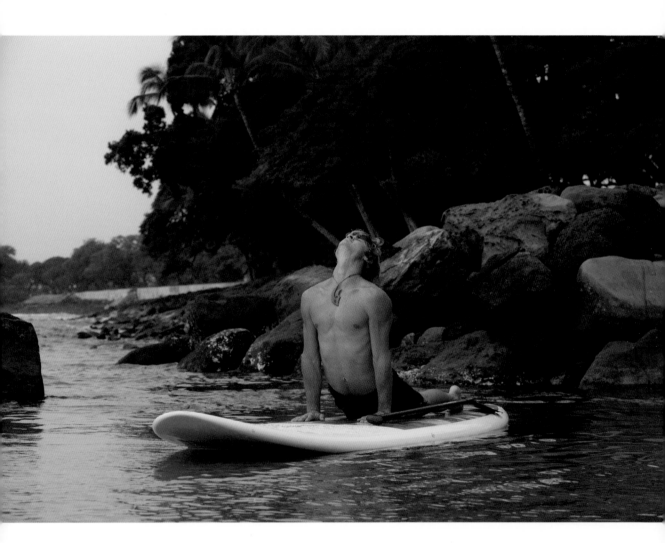

5. Standing Forward Bend with Shoulder Opener

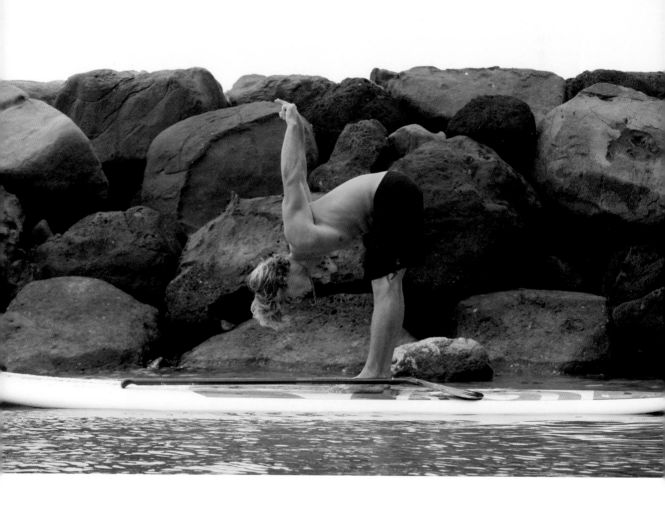

6. Standing Wrist Stretch

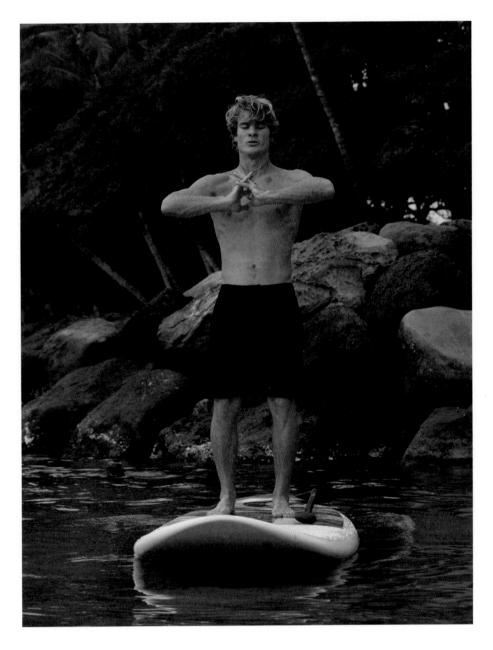

7. Mountain Pose with Prayer

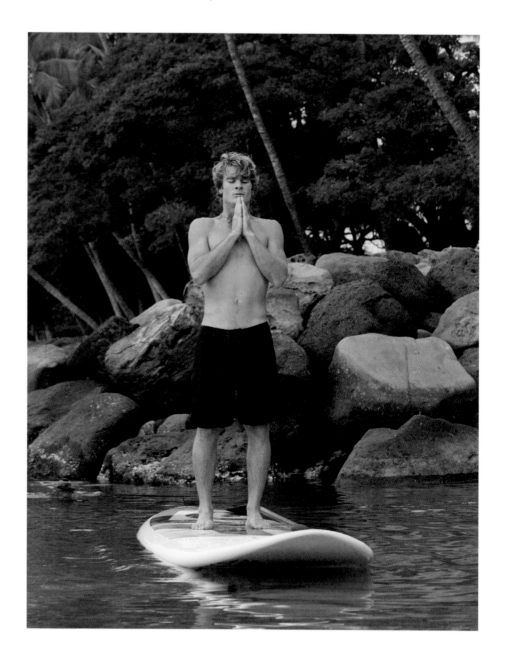

8. Standing Pigeon (aka Figure 4)

Standing pigeon opens the hips while creating balance.

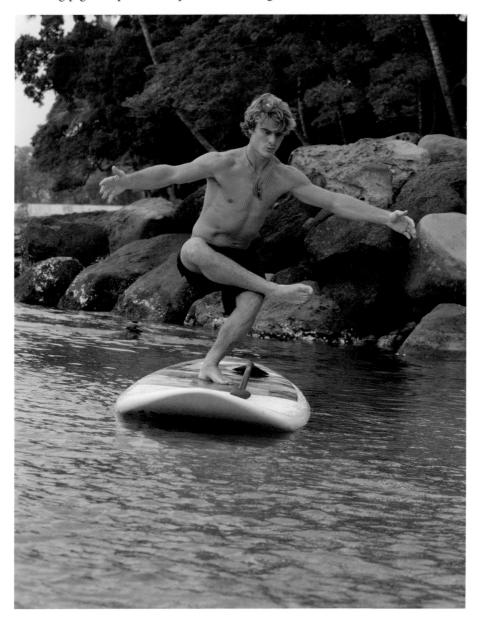

9. Headstand (Advanced Option)

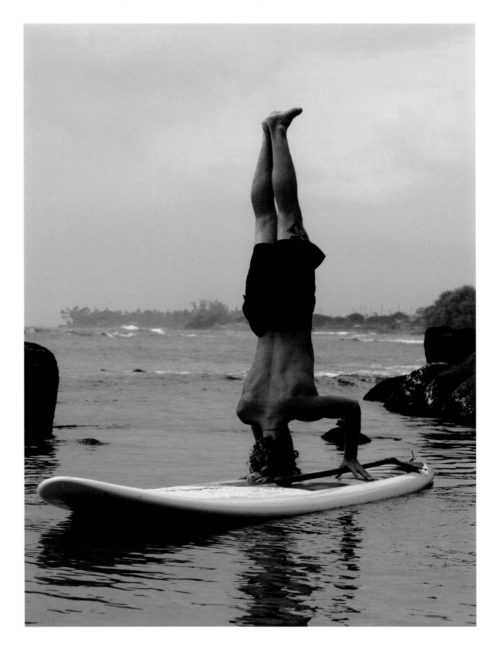

10. Standing Side Stretch with Paddle

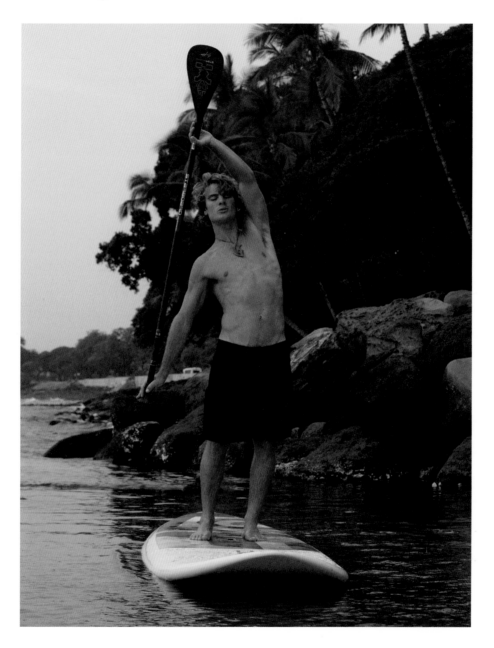

11. Beach Yoga: Butterfly with Shoulder Stretch

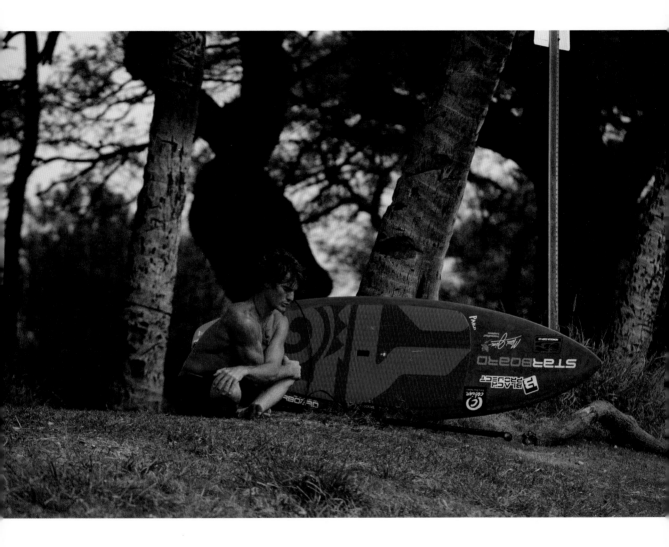

12. Beach Yoga: Wide Leg Side Stretch

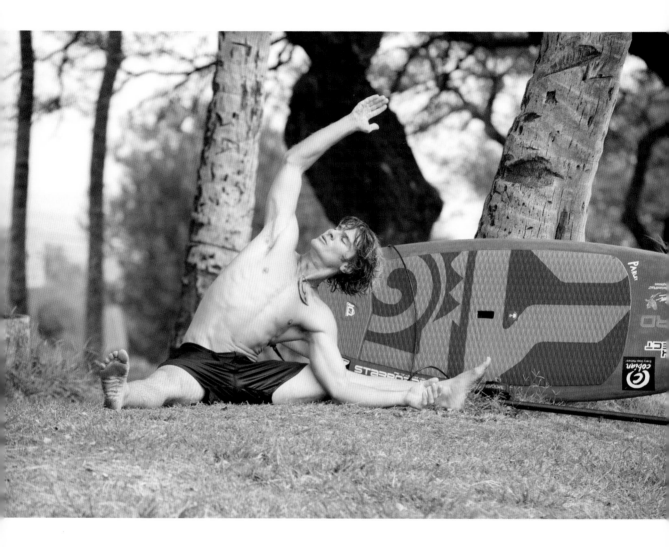

13. Beach Yoga: Pigeon

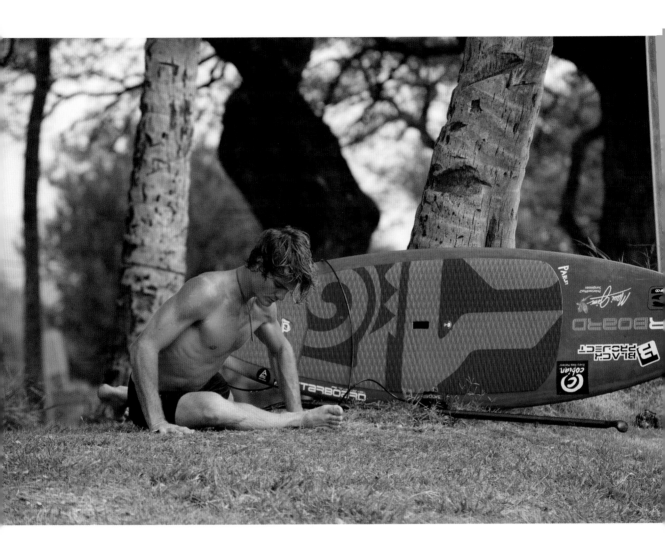

14. Beach Yoga: Staff Pose with Paddle

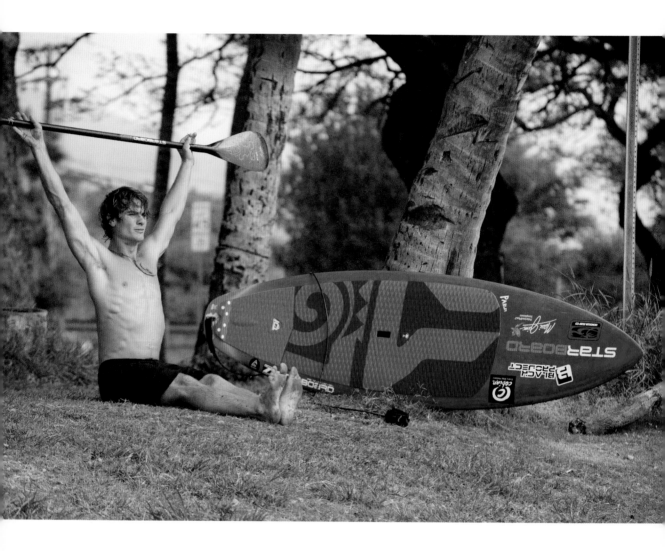

15. Beach Yoga: Seated Forward Bend

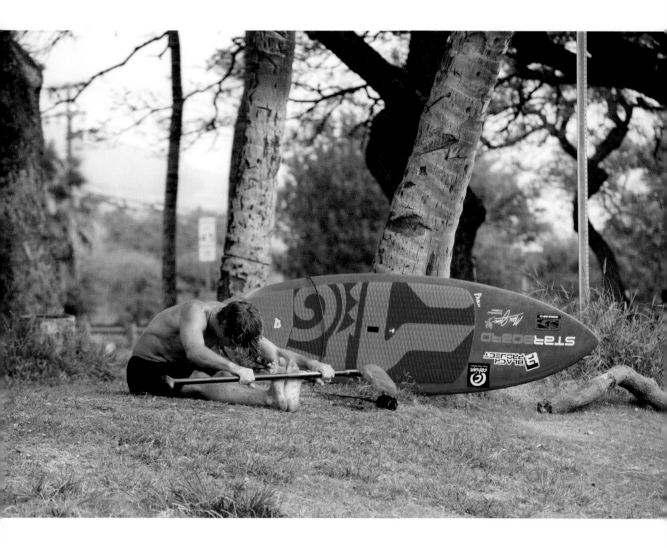

Zane's Tips to Help You Get More out of the Practice of Yoga and/or Surfing

- Wake up an hour earlier than you normally would and get comfortable with a routine you can follow, whether stretching, yoga, journaling, or a workout. This helps me feel less anxious and overwhelmed throughout my day, thus allowing me to be open to the "flow state."

- Practicing slackline has been a great way for me to connect my muscles and increase stability and strength before I hit the water. Learning how to slackline also gives you that state of flow, or at least will allow you to be more open to it throughout the day.

- Journaling first thing in the morning and at the end of the day has been beneficial for me to stay focused on the important things and has allowed me to move in a consistent direction. It has also allowed me to recognize and alter my state of mind—this opens the mind to opportunities of the flow state.

- Be open to the effects and benefits yoga may have, which will motivate you to be patient through the introduction to yoga.

Aloha and Mahalo, see you on the water!

> To be yourself in a world that is constantly trying to make you something else is the greatest accomplishment.
> —*Ralph Waldo Emerson*

FalconGuides Interview: Get to Know Zane Kekoa Schweitzer

Q. Who or what brought you into yoga to begin with? How did you get started and what got you hooked?

A. I first fell in love with yoga on my first trip to Japan. We were there for a windsurfing event, and I traveled with an older friend from Maui, as I was only fifteen years old and couldn't fly alone. Every day of that trip, Francisco would wake up before the sun came up and practice yoga in a traditional Japanese-style living room. I asked if I could join him, and it was history from there. After that trip to Japan learning yoga at fifteen years old, I recognized how important it is for a professional athlete and practiced often. As I grew up, I learned that there are so many more benefits to practicing yoga than just what a professional athlete might be looking for.

Q. What about surfing? How did that happen? Who, what, when, where, and why did you start and what has that journey been like?

A. I don't necessarily remember actually *learning* how to surf, as my parents brought me up on the front of their board and on the beach. My first surfing competition was when I was three years old; I won that event and I don't even remember it! But all I know is surfing has always been a part of my life and has created so many windows of opportunity for me solely by following my heart. Not to mention the connection I have found with nature through practicing a healthy, active lifestyle such as surfing from a young age.

Q. Can you describe your first or most transcendent experience with yoga? Anything that made you experience the flow state we are talking about in this book?

A. My first time ever feeling an effect from yoga, I wasn't old enough to realize I was altering my state of consciousness solely from breathing and stretching, All I knew was that it felt good and it was going to help my windsurfing for competition. I think a huge part of being able to experience these feeling with my first experience with yoga in Japan was because I was open to improvement, especially from someone I looked up to.

Q. What about surfing? Was there an experience that stands out more than the rest, and can you describe it in words? Where were you?

A. Similar to the effect with my first experience with yoga, I grew up always looking up to my dad, big brother, and friends because their lives revolved around the ocean and beach. Almost every time I go in the water, I feel what I now know as an altered state of consciousness. I feel like a young child, and any feelings of stress or negative emotions such as being overwhelmed or anxious seem to diminish.

Q. Are there specific places on earth where you feel most connected to this energy or flow state of consciousness, whether you are practicing yoga, surfing, both, or just being?

A. I feel this in many places around home in Hawaii, but I also feel I have many special connections to my environment around the world. At the top of my list are Tahiti, New Zealand, and the Basque country.

Q. Can you name your favorite surf break and where that is? What about for new surfers, is there a best place to learn in your opinion? Did you start with lessons or just go out and take the waves on? Is your family into surfing or were you a pioneer in your family?

A. My grandfather invented the sport of windsurfing, my father is an eighteen-time world champion, my little sister is a three-time national champion, and my brother is one of the best water sports videographers in the world. I myself dabble with a few world titles as well (fifteen individual world title events). Obviously our lives revolve around the ocean, for personal pleasure, family time, and/or as a competitive career. We also own a family business, Maui Sports Adventures, so we are grateful for the ocean and what it brings to us every day.

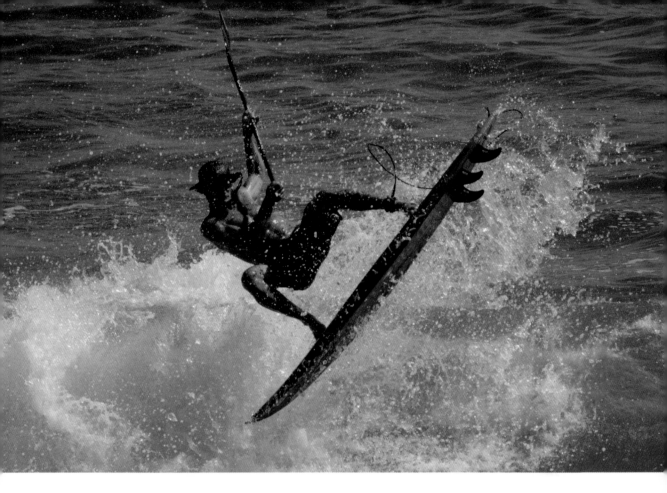

Q. Where and how did you start out in yoga? What was your first introduction to the practice and how do you suggest people start if they are considering getting into yoga? What is your favorite style to practice? Do you teach yoga? If so, what style?

A. For people looking to get into yoga and meditation, remember to be open to the benefits you'll receive, and hopefully this will allow you to be more patient and focus on breathing. What I have found by connecting with the ocean through sport is that I'm able to achieve this sense of altered consciousness, or "flow," as some people would call it, consistently just by being present in the moment while surfing, windsurfing, or stand-up paddling. I get the feeling that people who have practiced yoga for decades still may not experience this sense of flow as often as I do with so much of my time spent present in the moment on the water.

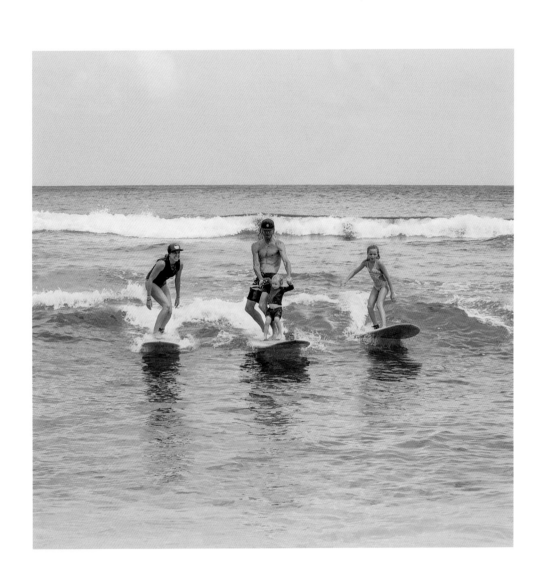

YOGI SURFING OCEAN MAMMA

Kendyl Beschen

When we enter into a flow state through yoga or surfing, we reintegrate with Spirit. This tunes us in to subtler frequencies, and we begin to see God in all things.
—*Kendyl*

About Kendyl

Kendyl is a forty-one-year-old mother of two and an avid surfer on the North Shore of Oahu. She has a master's degree in education and has been teaching music and Dharma Mittra Yoga classes on Oahu for about ten years. She also plays Hawaiian slack key guitar for yoga classes, events, and festivals and offers Reiki healing from her yurt in Pupukea. Her website is kendylmusicandyoga.com.

Kendyl's Yoga Practice

Note: Most of the poses that follow are advanced and should only be attempted by seasoned yoga practitioners.

1. Kapiasana (Cresent Lunge)

Come into a deep lunge. Interlace fingers in kali mudra (steeple grip) and inhale the arms up. Use the bind of the hands to pull your biceps behind your ears. Lift the heart. Engage mula bandha (root lock) to draw energy up the spine. Follow your breath and stay still. This pose helps open your hips, chest, lungs, and shoulders.

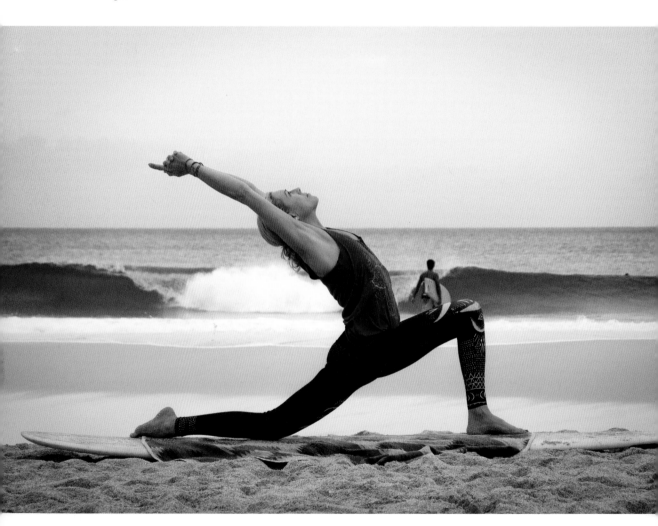

2. Kapiasana (Crescent Lunge with Bind)

Extend the right arm back and take the inside of the right foot. Begin working the foot toward the inside of the right elbow and connect your hands behind your head. With consistent practice you will be able to make the bind. This pose strengthens the entire body and improves balance and concentration.

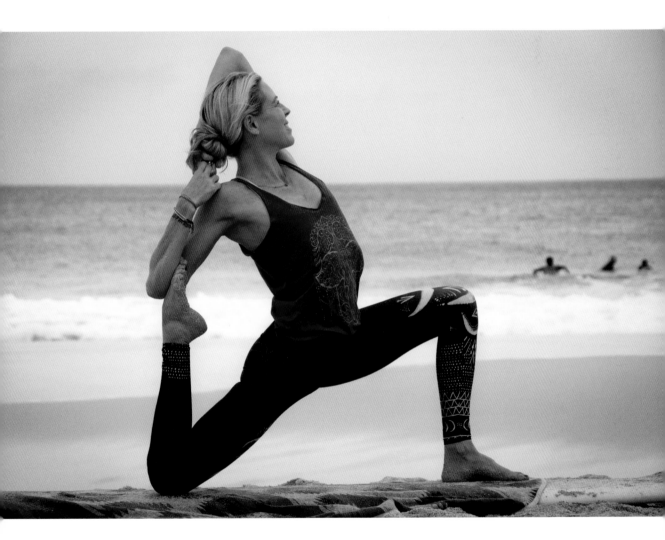

3. Eka Pada Koundinyasana II (Split-Legged Arm Balance)

Release the crescent lunge and move into a "leg over arm lunge." Bring your right arm under your right leg to create a shelf for the leg. Place your right leg over the right upper arm and experiment with lifting the right foot off the ground. Then lift the left leg as well. This fun arm balance tones the belly and spine and strengthens the arms and wrists.

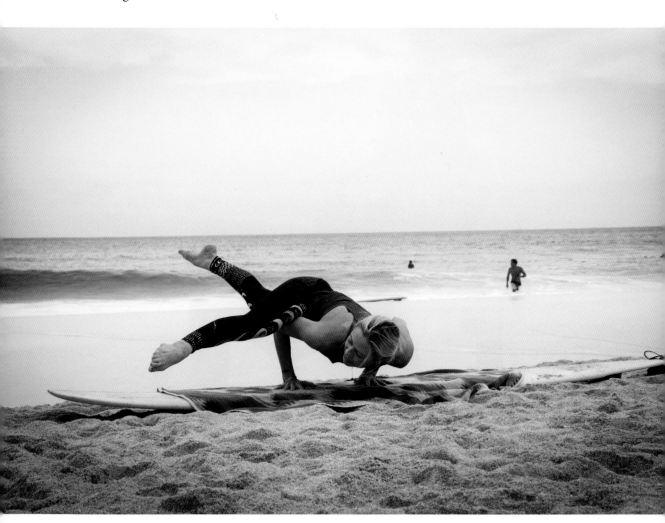

4. Parivrtta Parsvakonasana (Revolved Side Angle Pose)

Begin from a high lunge with right leg forward. Draw your belly toward your spine as you twist your torso to bring your left arm to the outside of your right thigh. Connect hands in a prayer position or take a bind looking over your right shoulder. This deep twist challenges balance and strengthens legs and core. It also helps detoxify the body by wringing out impurities and stimulating fresh blood flow through the organs.

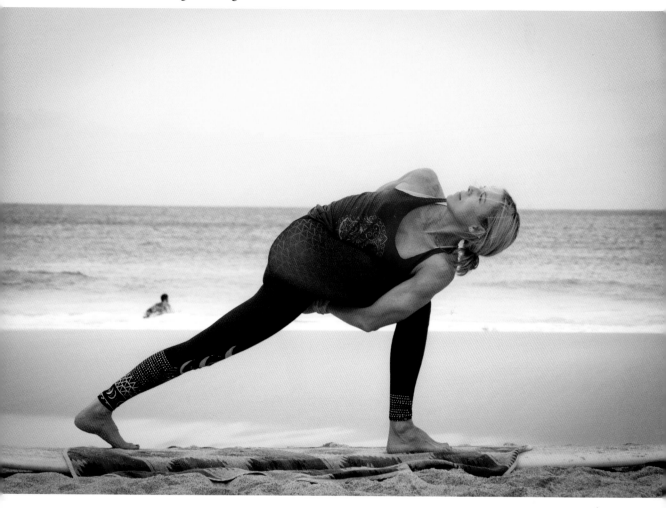

5. Eka Pada Galavasana (Flying Pigeon)

Begin by taking deep calming breaths in pigeon pose to open the hip and prepare for the flying pigeon arm balance. If the hip has opened enough, hook the top of your right foot around your left upper arm. Engage uddiyana bandha (abdominal lift) by pulling the belly up and in. Shift your upper body forward and shoot the left leg behind you to create a counterbalance. This pose strengthens the arms and core and stretches the hips and legs.

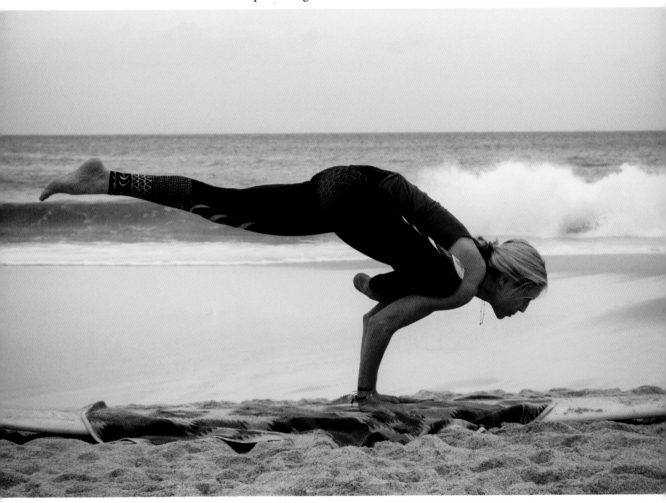

6. Svarga Dvijasana (Bird of Paradise Pose)

Start from extended side angle pose (utthita parsvakonasana) with the right leg in front. Bind by reaching your right arm underneath your right leg and your left arm behind your back. Look down at your right foot and bring your left foot to meet it. Shift weight onto the left leg and slowly make your way up to standing. Engage mula bandha and uddiyana bandha to steady yourself; gradually straighten your right leg, eventually bringing it into full extension.

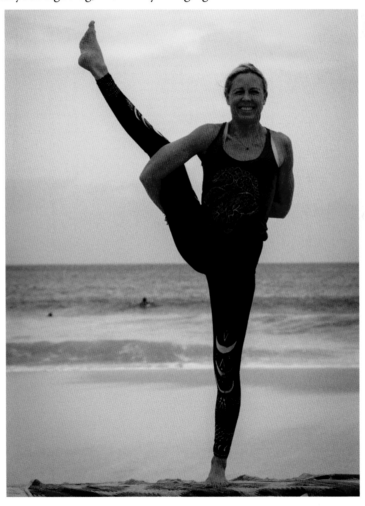

7. Shirsasana with Padmasana (Headstand with Lotus)

Grab hold of opposite elbows so that your elbows are directly under your shoulders. With your head on the mat, interlace your fingers and place them around your head like a helmet. Walk your hips over your shoulders and carefully bring thighs to the chest. If you have the balance, extend your knees up and eventually straighten the legs. If you have a lotus pose, you can bring your legs to lotus and stay still, concentrating on the space between your eyebrows. Fresh oxygenated blood flows to the brain.

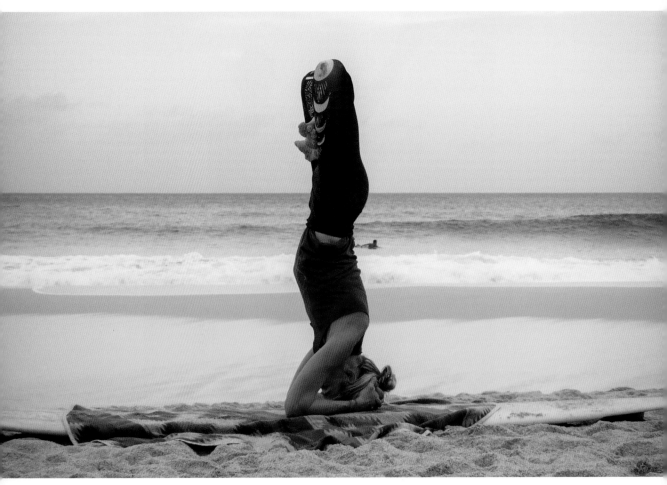

8. Halasana (Plow Pose)

Begin lying flat on your back and lift your legs and hips up toward the ceiling. Bring your torso perpendicular to the ground and slowly lower your legs behind your head. If your toes don't touch the floor, support your back with your hands.

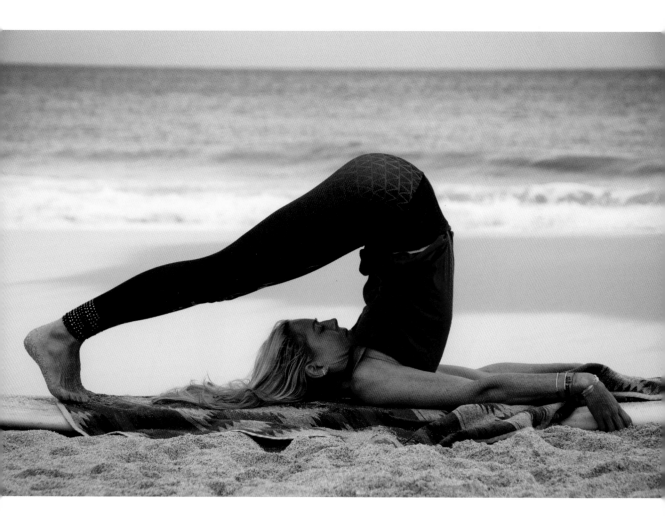

9. Urdhva Dhanurasana (Upward Bow Pose)

Begin lying flat on your back and bring your heels about hip-width apart close to your butt. Place your hands back by your ears. Lift your head off the floor, push through the feet, and straighten your arms as much as possible. This energizing heart-opener stretches the chest and lungs while toning the arms, legs, butt, belly, and spine. It also stimulates the vagus nerve, thyroid, and pituitary glands.

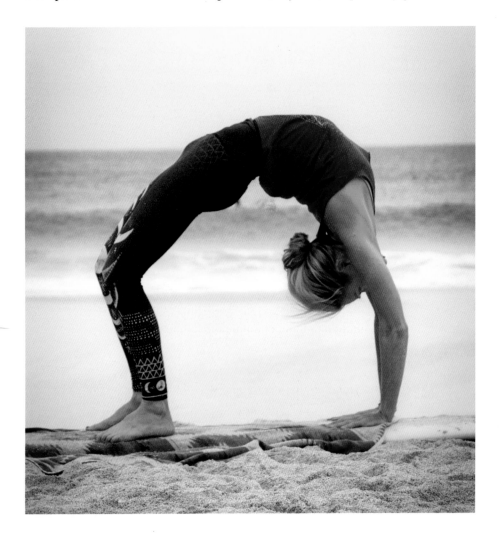

10. Paschimottanasana (Seated Forward Fold)

Bend your knees and link your chest to your thighs. Knees can stay bent to protect the lower back. With each inhalation, lift and lengthen the torso; with each exhalation release a little more fully into the forward bend. This calming pose stretches the spine, shoulders, and hamstrings while stimulating the digestive organs.

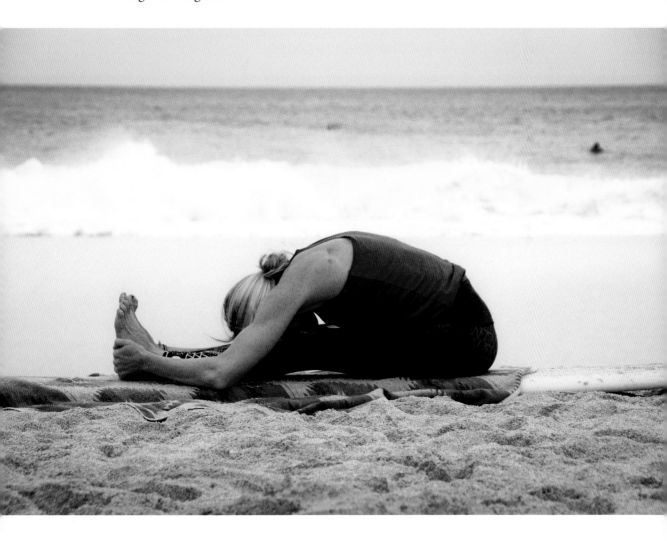

Kendyl's Tips to Help You Get More out of the Practice of Yoga and/or Surfing

My best advice for readers is to let go of ego and allow yourselves to enjoy the learning process. Every yogi and every surfer has to go through the beginner phase. If we are kind to ourselves, we can laugh at ourselves when we fall, and get back up and try again until we find our flow.

We learn by example, so seek out good teachers and do as they do.

Yoga and surfing are spiritual practices, so if you approach them with reverence and a pure heart, you will find what you are looking for.

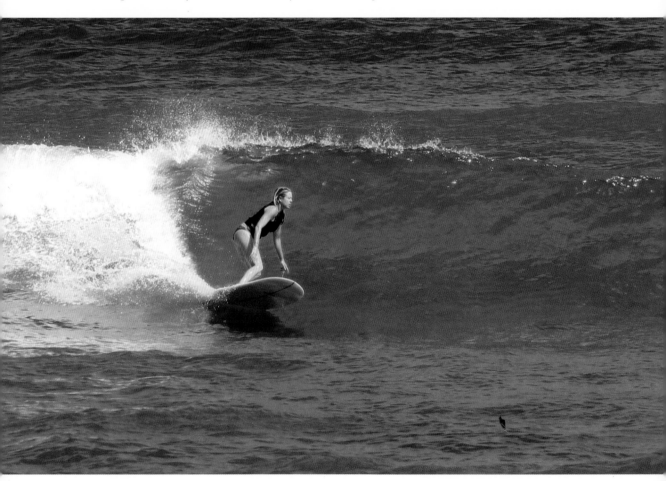

FalconGuides Interview: Get to Know Kendyl Beschen

Q. Who or what brought you into yoga to begin with? How did you get started and what got you hooked?

A. I began practicing yoga when I was pregnant with my first child. Before that time, I was teaching elementary school, and like many people I felt I was too busy for yoga. If I had any free time, I just wanted to surf! But, of course, pregnancy made me slow down, and my belly got so big that I didn't feel comfortable surfing. The pregnancy forced me to tune in to what was going on inside my body. I started reading books about yoga and began doing prenatal yoga DVDs. I learned how stretching helped my awkward body release tension, and I discovered that breathing and meditation techniques helped me feel more peaceful and relax for deeper sleep. I was very receptive to the ancient teachings of yoga because I felt that they were helping me make my body a healthy home for my growing child.

Q. What about surfing? How did that happen? Who, what, when, where, and why did you start and what has that journey been like?

A. I grew up in San Clemente, California. Surfing was a large part of our town's culture, yet when I was young, hardly any girls surfed. A couple of my friends and I were recruited by our track coach to help start a girls surfing team. At first we were so bad it was embarrassing, but we had a lot of fun out in the ocean together! We encouraged each other to keep trying, and luckily we lived near San Onofre, which has one of the best learning waves in the world. I remember when everything finally came together for us and we were able to ride those long, slow San-O waves all the way to the beach. It was the most exhilarating feeling, and we were hooked for life. My deep love for the ocean led me to Hawaii when I was nineteen, and I have been surfing in this glorious turquoise water ever since.

Q. Can you describe your first or most transcendent experience with yoga? Anything that made you experience the flow state we are talking about in this book?

A. I found my first real yoga teacher about eleven years ago. I had recently given birth to my first child and was recovering from an emergency C-section. I arrived at her class feeling injured, off-balance, overweight, and literally leaking breast milk. My teacher was a beautiful Brazilian woman who reminded me of an Amazonian warrioress. She was so strong and fierce, yet she had the most peaceful energy. I wanted to be in her presence, and I wanted to become more like her! I started going to her classes whenever I had free time, even if it meant I went to yoga instead of surfing. I knew the yoga was helping me so much, and I began to see rapid progress in my practice, as I did whatever my teacher told me to do. I would sweat and cry and leave the studio feeling like a new woman and a better mother.

Q. What about surfing? Was there an experience that stands out more than the rest, and can you describe it in words? Where were you?

A. Everything came together for me when I begin surfing daily in Hawaii and really got to connect to the spirit of Mother Ocean. I liked surfing in California, but the water was cold and sometimes polluted. The water in Hawaii is clean, clear, and filled with life. I felt at one with the colorful fish, whales, dolphins, turtles, and living reef. Surfing became less of a sport and more of a spirit dance with nature.

Q. Are there specific places on earth where you feel most connected to this energy or flow state of consciousness, whether you are practicing yoga, surfing, both, or just being?

A. The North Shore of Oahu is definitely a vortex of energy. Waves of energy are literally drawn here like a magnet with extreme power and force. Rainbows are everywhere, and plants and animals thrive in this lush and abundantly rich environment. My yoga teacher comes to visit me sometimes, and she always talks about the energy here and how it is so powerful. This power and the force in this vortex naturally makes many people more receptive to spirit. We become more in tune with our earth element. We become more reverent and humbler, which allows us to access the flow states of consciousness through yoga and surfing.

I have seen beginning surfers and yogis get a taste of the magical "flow state." That's how we all get hooked! With consistent practice this state becomes natural and spontaneous. We have five types of waves in our brains: gamma, beta, alpha, theta, and delta. Each frequency serves a purpose, but in these fast-paced digital days most people are overstimulated and gamma and beta waves dominate. When we do things like ride a wave or get deep into a yoga/pranayama/meditation practice, we tune in to our alpha waves, and maybe even into our theta and delta waves. These magical waves promote a sense of well-being, deep healing, and pure creativity.

Q. Can you name your favorite surf break and where that is? What about for new surfers, is there a best place to learn in your opinion? Did you start with

lessons or just go out and take the waves on? Is your family into surfing or were you a pioneer in your family?

A. My eleven-year-old daughter and I surf all over the North Shore year-round. She is getting really good, and I love watching her giggle and sing as she paddles out and dances on her waves. When it's small in the summertime, we longboard Laniakea, Chuns, Kammieland, or Backyards. We practice cross-stepping and riding the nose of our longboards. The small summer waves break close to the reef, and since the water is more still, we often are able to see eagle rays, reef sharks, and large schools of tropical fish. In the spring and fall we enjoy Rocky Point, Pupukea, and Sunset Beach. The waves are fast and fun, and we often surf with other moms and kids. During the large winter swells on the North Shore we often surf Freddy Land, Pua'ena Point, and Melaekahana. These waves are "reforms," meaning they break first on an outer reef and lose some power, so they are not as strong when they break the second time. These are great waves for learning because beginners can catch the whitewash and still have plenty of time to stand up and ride the wave for a long time.

Q. Where and how did you start out in yoga? What was your first introduction to the practice and how do you suggest people start if they are considering getting into yoga? What is your favorite style to practice? Do you teach yoga? If so, what style?

A. My first real yoga teacher touched my heart and soul. She was a disciple of Sri Dharma Mittra and led playful, yet very spiritual classes. She taught me to stand on my head for long periods of time and have compassion for all beings. She showed me the path of the peaceful warrior, which was exactly what I needed as a new mother. I completed my Life of a Yogi Teacher Training Program with Sri Dharma Mittra in New York City in 2009. I taught and studied at Dharma Yoga Los Angeles under my mentor, Sonya Enchill, for about a year and have been teaching on the North Shore since 2010. A lot of surfers, including a handful of professional surfers, regularly take my classes. I actually just finished my second year teaching a monthlong workshop for one of the surf teams competing in the Pipeline Backdoor Shootout. Yoga is so good for athletes, and it is such a joy to share the practice with them. I teach Dharma Yoga, which is a classical Hatha Raja yoga practice. Dharma is almost eighty-eight years old, and he is so vibrantly healthy and happy. I pass on his teachings to the best of my ability.

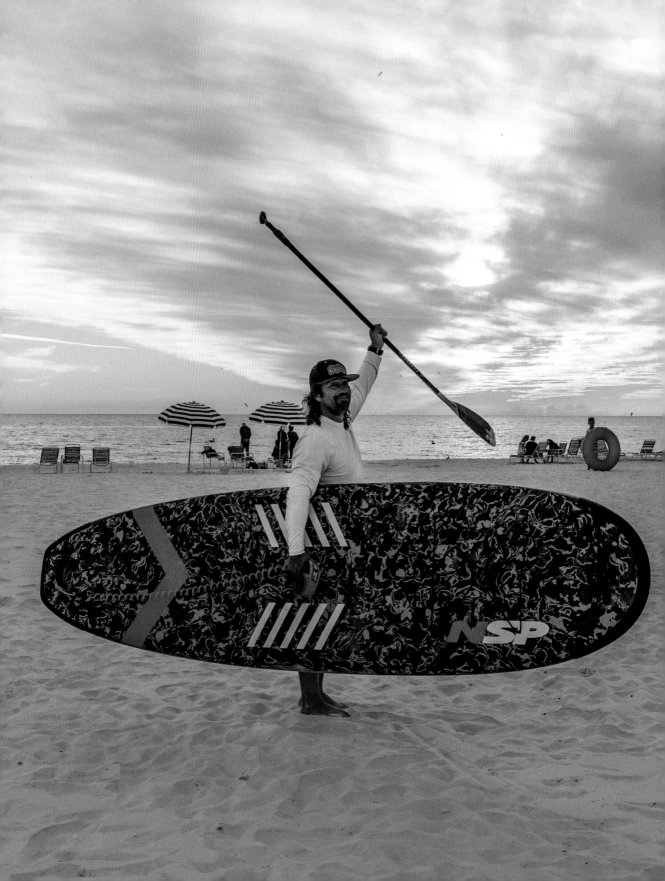

SUP SURF YOGA
Jeramie Vaine

And, when you want something, all the universe conspires in helping you to achieve it.

—*Paulo Coelho*, The Alchemist

About Jeramie

Jeramie is a traveler, lover of all things water, a student, and a teacher with a passion to grow as much as humanly possible. After years of wakeboarding, stand-up paddleboarding, and yoga, he was introduced to combined SUP and yoga in 2011. He received his CorePower Yoga 200-hour Power Yoga teaching certification in 2014. Today he is a Surftech and NSP North America team manager and SUP and SUP yoga instructor, sharing his passions of teaching and the water and connecting with people around the globe, whether through direct contact at Wanderlust Festivals, stand-up paddleboard events, workshops, and trainings, or through a virtual connection of writing, blogging, and social media.

Find Jeramie on Instagram at @jvaine1.

Jeramie's Yoga for Surfing Routine

The practices that help me get to that flow state are not something we can Google. It requires us to begin to believe and do. The following practices I have broken down in importance for me. But we are all different. As long as we are out practicing or surfing, we are that much closer to finding that energy, that state. Meditation has joined my routine over the past few years. But it has taken work and an understanding. It started simply as breathing and has now blossomed into a form of its own. Whether I'm starting the day, getting ready for bed, paddling out into the surf, or diving down below the surface of the water, it is meditation that helps me. I start with cleansing breaths with deep exhales—just five of them. Then repeat until the mind wants to wander off. And then sit. Acknowledge that the thoughts are just thoughts—not good or bad. Dismiss them.

Another great way to stay in this place is to connect with words that help keep you grounded or connected. I often use ones that resonate with my mood or current feeling that day—love, opportunity, happiness. Those are on my inhale. And on the exhale—ego, attachment, anger. There are many other ways to venture out into the world of meditation. But these have worked for me. Joining a guided meditation is always a great place to open the mind to the world of meditation as well.

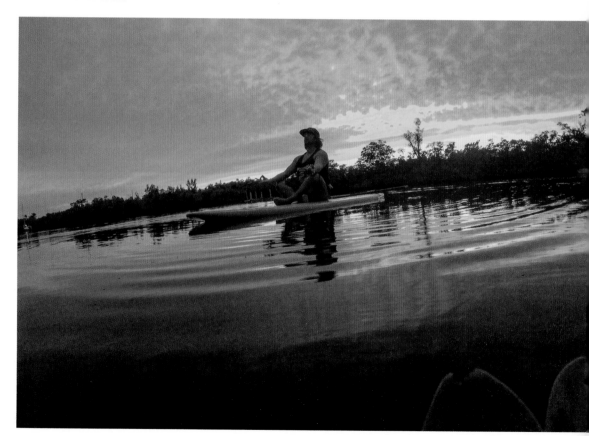

Jeramie's Yoga for Surfers Flow

This sequence can be for beginners or advanced yoga practitioners. It is my go-to sequence, whether for a warm-up or conditioning.

1. Chair Pose

Start in chair pose with feet grounded down through all four corners. Knees are bent and just behind the toes and in line with the toes. Try not to let them splay open to the sides. Arms rise above. If the shoulders are tight, open the arms wider, then bring the shoulders back into the joint.

On the exhale, bring your hands down to the shins or ground in forward fold.

On the inhale, rise up to flatten the back and lengthen through the back of the legs in halfway lift. Peer over the edge of the mat to help create this space.

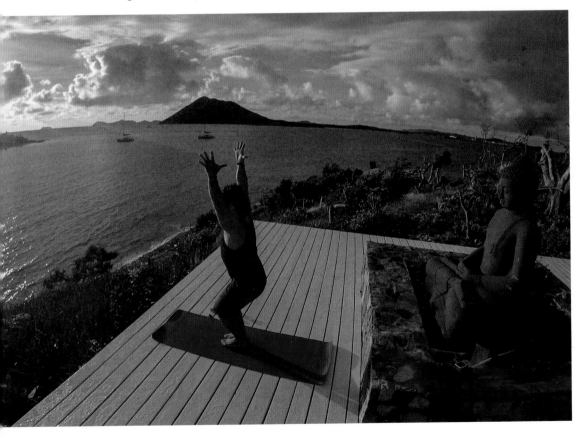

2. Crow

Crow or crane pose is our next stop. Plant the palms. Bring the knees onto the back of the triceps. Keep the toes connected to the earth. Begin to hinge forward so the shoulders are over the fingertips. Engage the core and slowly float one toe off the mat. Then place it back on the ground and float the other. Work on getting hang time with each toe. In time both toes will float off the earth. Trust that you can hold yourself.

From crow move into a high plank, then lower down through chaturanga.

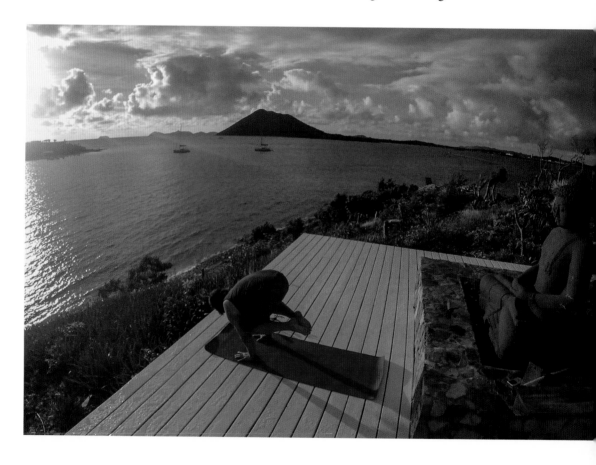

3. Upward-Facing Dog

Lay the toes flat on the mat, pull the hands toward the body, and move into upward-facing dog.

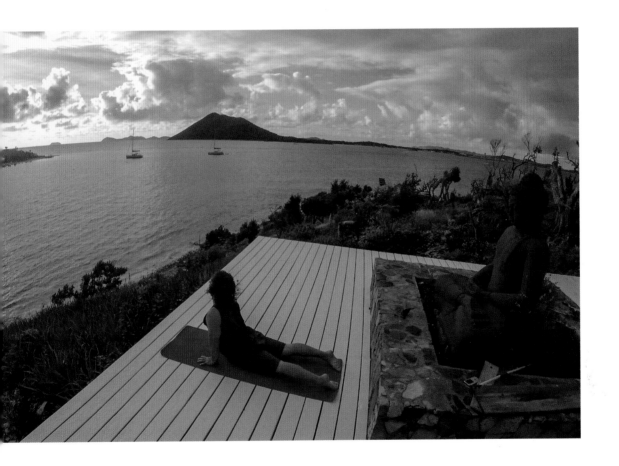

4. Down Dog

Press back to downward-facing dog.

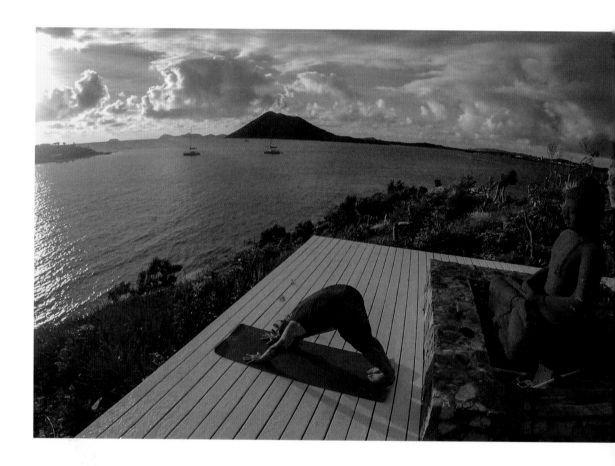

5. Crescent Lunge

Bring the right leg forward so the right pinky toe is just inside of the thumb. Look at the knee to make sure it is behind the ankle. If your balance is unstable, drop the left knee to the earth. Otherwise, ground down through the left ball of the foot and the right foot. Engage the core and rise up. Hands can rise straight up. Or drop them down in a 90-degree bend, gently lift the chin, and gaze upward.

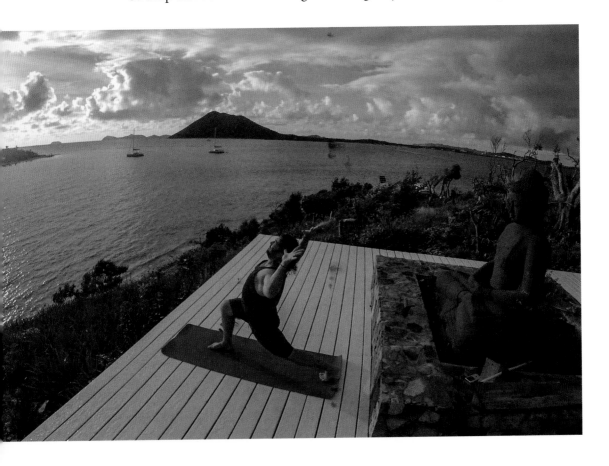

6. Lunge Twist

From crescent lunge, with the knee dropped or up, depending on balance, plant the left hand under the left shoulder. Raise the right hand high to the sky. The feet stay in the same place. The twist comes from the core. Try to resist the urge to rest on your stomach.

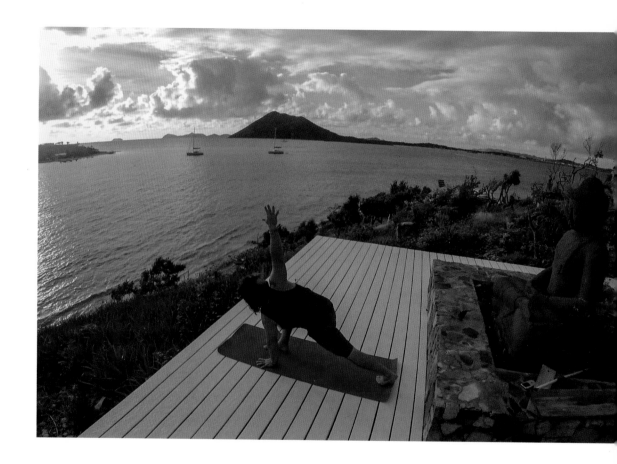

7. Wild Thing

Wild thing is also called flipping the dog. Start from side plank, either full expression or on the knees. Roll the right arm open and back toward the ground. The right toes will find the ground and then the foot will plant. Roll back over to high plank. Lower down, chaturanga, and press to upward-facing dog, then to downward-facing dog. Then side plank onto the left leg. Repeat the whole sequence on this side.

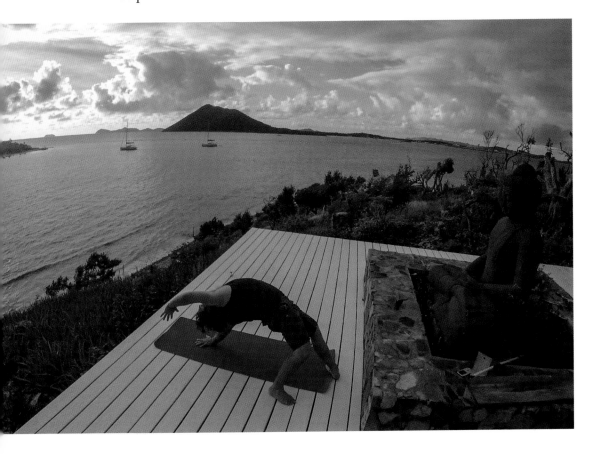

Jeramie's Tips for Yoga and Surfing Success
Connect with the Water

This is one of the things I enjoy doing to slow myself down and start the process of connection. Before putting my leash on, I walk over to the water, dip my toes or hands into the waves, and take a moment to be still. My breath is natural, and my gaze drifts over the water and my surroundings. I check in with my body and my mind. I look to see if I am bringing anything extraneous with me to this sanctuary. And some days I am. This is when I resort to meditation and work on letting go of anything I am holding on to. The reason is multifaceted but simply put: If my mind is not right, my time on the water will suffer. And that defeats the entire purpose. We have all been there before, fighting a battle inside our head, missing out on the beauty that is directly in front of us. Use the meditation practice I mentioned earlier to surrender to the surrounding. It has been extremely helpful and beneficial in making my time on the water a great one. Learn from others. This is one of the most important parts of my practice now. Before I was always nervous to take a lesson or join a class. But now each time I step into the studio with a new teacher or take a lesson in paddling or surfing, the lessons reveal themselves in larger ways.

There always is a takeaway that taps into my personal life and then transitions into my world of surfing, teaching, and yoga.

Surf with People

This sounds simple, but I love to surround myself with good friends while on the water. The level of excitement is heightened and so is the ability to connect with the flow state. Each wave I take has not only excitement but friends sharing in that excitement. It is like a multiplier to the flow state. And what is better than paddling back out and hearing a great friend hooting and hollering because they are as excited as you are, if not more. We all want to receive the maximum benefit from whatever we do. It is the same for our practice on and off the water.

Things I Try to Keep in Mind on My Mat or Out on the Water

1. I made it to this place. And I am grateful that my body, mind, soul, and the universe have allowed it to happen.

2. Connection with the breath and our surroundings. Even though we've made it to the water, it doesn't mean that our mind will not wander off to that nagging to-do list or that phone call we are supposed to have.

3. Be open to having a not-so-great practice or session. Look for the lesson and experience that presented itself. Maybe the set waves disappeared, or every pose was a struggle. But you had a conversation with a new or old friend or saw something made you smile. Find the takeaway that truly makes you smile.

FalconGuides Interview: Get to Know Jeramie Vaine

Q. Who or what brought you into yoga to begin with? How did you get started and what got you hooked?

A. My love for the water is where it all started. Working with Paddleboard Orlando, in central Florida, I was introduced to a beautiful community of humans. During the classes we played around with some yoga poses. But that was the extent of my yoga practice until one day after paddling. A friend asked, "Why don't you come to yoga tonight?" I was apprehensive, but on a Tuesday night in October I walked through the doors of Guruv Yoga. Thirty-plus yoga mats were neatly laid on the floor, some with students sitting or practicing, others vacant. My friend assisted me in finding a spot. And just like catching that first wave, my emotions started to drift away as soon as my body began to move. It was a challenging class that left me dripping with sweat and smiling from ear to ear. And I instantly signed up for more classes. During class the teacher, Tymi Howard, who is now my mentor, would always offer room to play. My fellow students would float through handstand or some other means of balancing on their hands or forearms. And I attempted to join in. Some things were attainable; others still remain a goal. But I needed more. It began to fill a void in my world. Living in central Florida, I made my way to the ocean a few times a week. Some days the surf was there and others not so much. I craved that freedom and flow pushing myself to places that push me outside my comfort zone. And the excitement that comes along with knowing anything is possible if I just try, believe, and do. And to this day, it is why I head to my mat.

Q. What about surfing? How did that happen? Who, what, when, where, and why did you start and what has that journey been like?

A. Growing up surrounded by freshwater, the idea of surfing always excited me. But it was through a longer roundabout that surfing entered my life. Wakeboarding played a larger part in my life—competing, teaching, traveling. One of the trips brought me to South Carolina to teach, which is where I met a dear friend,

Ken Hall, who passed along his passion of surfing. I was eighteen years old when I caught my first wave. During the summer we made daily trips to the beach, sometimes just to watch and learn about the ocean and how the waves work. Other times we paddled out. Over the few months I called Charleston home, I probably caught about ten waves. But it solidified a spot in my life and a connection with the ocean, one that would lie dormant until my early thirties.

Q. Can you describe your first or most transcendent experience with yoga? Anything that made you experience the flow state we are talking about in this book?

A. My mind was racing all day—and not in a good way. I was worrying about a recent breakup, financial troubles, and what was next in my life. I dragged myself to yoga, almost turning around twice. During class I moved through the poses. My mind would wander off and I'd find myself lost. It wasn't until we headed into savasana that a simple cue—roll the head from side to side—triggered something. All the things I held on to so tightly released. And I slipped into the most peaceful savasana for what felt like hours. On the drive home, a feeling of euphoria overtook my body. And it was at this moment that my life began to change. I began to look at the world differently. There were no more obstacles preventing me from doing what I wanted, just ways to overcome the minor bumps in the road that I once viewed as obstacles. This experience reconnected my world to days I had on the water. Viewing challenges in a new light and creating that excitement to overcome everything. This feeling continues to reappear throughout my practice. Some days it is in challenging poses and transitions, and other times in meditation. I now have a deeper understanding about it. It was there during my childhood and teenage years wakeboarding and playing hockey. It also exposed me to the power of yoga. If I could make it to my mat when life threw obstacles my way, I had a way to ground and put myself in a place to work through them.

Q. What about surfing? Was there an experience that stands out more than the rest, and can you describe it in words? Where were you?

A. Every day I paddle out, the ocean always provides a lesson. But there have been a few occasions where I experienced the flow state that I felt in yoga. During a contest in Santa Cruz, California, we had the opportunity to surf a world-class spot. On this day the waves arrived and showed why it wears the name "Steamer Lane." As we paddled out, the swell began to peak. With the sounding of the horn, the heat started. And moments later the set of the day did too—eight to ten waves. With my heart racing and adrenaline rushing, I paddled into the second wave. But as I looked down the line, I pulled off, which was a mistake. As I turned around to set up for the next one, the biggest wave of the set appeared and was already breaking. As I dove down deep, that feeling arose. I knew I could handle this and get through. After what felt like a few seconds, I paddled back out and caught a few waves before the heat ended. But what actually happened was that I was caught inside for over ten minutes, taking wave after wave on the head. But that feeling kept me calm and in control.

About a year and a half earlier, "Big Wednesday" hit Southern California. Record-setting surf pounded the coast. Two friends, Morgan Hoesterey and George Plsek, and I set out to catch a few of these waves. Paddling out was a bit of a struggle. I made it through the beach break and gazed over to see Morgan coming down the face of a monster wave. As I paddled over to her, that feeling once again began to take over. Before I made it to her, a set appeared outside. I waited and paddled into a left with speed, adrenaline, and focus. There was no question of not making it. The raw power and energy of Mother Ocean connected with me, allowing me to move with ease and grace as if I had rehearsed this moment for years.

Q. Are there specific places on earth where you feel most connected to this energy or flow state of consciousness, whether you are practicing yoga, surfing, both, or just being?

A. The connection with water is something that I've felt for years. As my yoga practice has grown, the feeling of connection has deepened. Over the years stand-up paddling has opened my eyes to all the possibilities of enjoying the power of nature. Rivers, oceans, lakes, and even pools. Visiting any one of these bodies of water, I take time to sit and listen and feel the surroundings. Time seems to drifts away. The mind calms. During these moments, whether long or brief, the connection begins to deepen. It truly is something that I struggle to describe because each setting is so unique. But that feeling is so familiar. The one that has led me back to my mat and onto the water.

Q. Can you name your favorite surf break and where that is? What about for new surfers, is there a best place to learn in your opinion? Did you start with lessons or just go out and take the waves on? Is your family into surfing or were you a pioneer in your family?

A. As with my yoga practice my favorite spot has slowly evolved. Now it's the place where I have the most enjoyable time on the water. It may not host the best waves or the biggest. The overall experience is most important. Time spent with good friends, whether new or old, with lots of laughs and smiles. This "place" has appeared in a multitude of locations—warm tropical board-short sessions, snowy gray wetsuit-clad days—on rivers and lakes. When it all comes together, the physical location is removed. But the experience is what leaves the lasting mark. How do we go about finding these experiences? The first step is getting out on the water.

Lessons are always a great way to share the experience. Being out in the water with someone who understands this feeling will help flatten out the learning curve. And they will have the knowledge of the perfect place to learn. Surfing can be intimidating. And Mother Ocean can hide her teeth. The guidance of a teacher, whether a friend, surf school, or private lesson, will help you stay out of that dangerous place and in the fun zone. Growing up in central New England, the ocean was always in my life, but surfing was not. Sports like ice hockey and waterskiing filled the void until that day my friend brought me out to surf. It was a lesson on life and understanding my surroundings. Having the gentle guidance of Ken Hall close by softened the edges. To this day I am beyond grateful that I had him there as a mentor and friend.

Q. Where and how did you start out in yoga? What was your first introduction to the practice and how do you suggest people start if they are considering getting into yoga? What is your favorite style to practice? Do you teach yoga? If so, what style?

A. Surfing or yoga—both can be so intimidating to start. Our mind always tries to convince us of the worst possible outcome, and usually it is successful in doing so. So the first step is mentally preparing ourselves. We can do this, whether the experience is trying or amazing. There are so many great studios and classes offered. But the perfect one is the one that gets us through the doors and on our mat. For me, I was surrounded by amazing people who encouraged me to keep trying things. Yoga was one of them. It started because I tried stand-up paddle-boarding. Then it was an introduction to yoga. Hot yoga, power yoga—it was all I wanted to do. My mentor, Tymi Howard of Guruv Yoga in Orlando, said to me, "There are seven more limbs of the yogic tree. And you soon will understand them." I'll never forget those words.

I completed my teacher training in CorePower Yoga in Southern California. My view on yoga started to change. Today I've slowed it down—meditation, yin, restorative, and beginner yoga. The reason behind the change was me listening to my body, letting it be my guide, not the mind. The words from Tymi still echo in the back of my head. Teaching has solidified a passion in my life to empower others to try something new. The classes I teach vary from all-level SUP yoga to restorative yoga for athletes. The goal is to reach one person, just as my mentor did for me.

Q. Do you feel a beginner can access the feeling of the flow state either in yoga or surfing, or would you say it's more of an advanced practice that they can work their way up to with consistent dedicated practice?

A. The flow state feeling is something that any and all can experience. But the mind is the key piece. If you are guarded or put up walls, the process is inhibited. So we must be open to experience anything and everything. Many of us seek the flow state. And when we seek it, it often avoids us because we are not in the moment and not in the experience. Even experienced practitioners and surfers who know of the flow state may not experience it for years. But a new student with an open, experienced mind can have the flow state visit them on the first day.

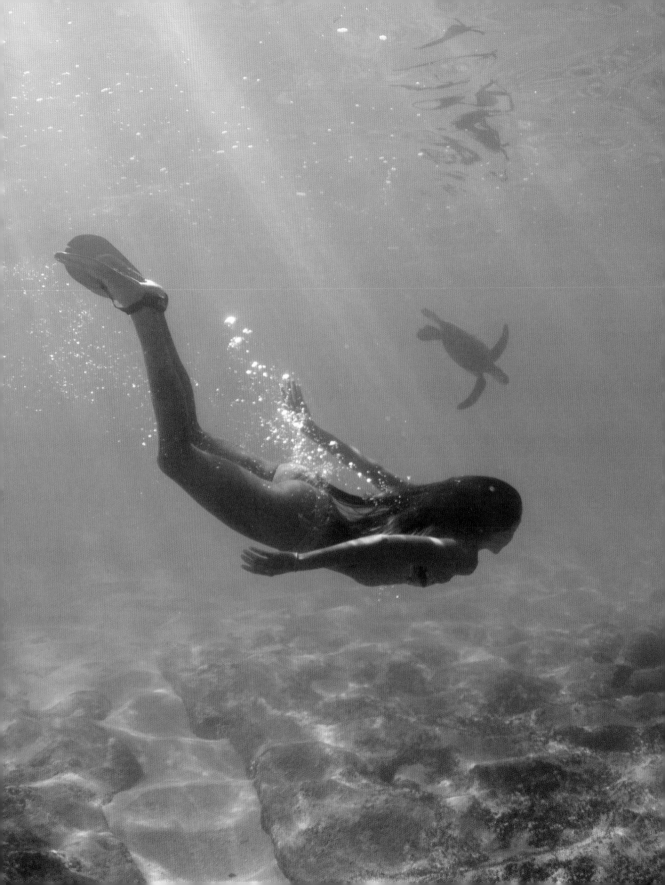

YOGA FOR HAPPINESS
Noelani Love

Only love is real.
—*MC Yogi*

About Noelani

Hailing from the North Shore of Oahu in Hawaii, Noelani Love brings soft melodies and her sweet ukulele sounds to the yoga and spiritual music world. Noelani finds much of her inspiration in nature: surfing, practicing yoga, songwriting, free diving, and designing jewelry. Finding her voice as a young mother has been instrumental in her development as a singer and teacher to empower many to live out their dreams.

As a trained doula and yoga teacher in kundalini, vinyasa, and mantra, Noelani teaches a blend of these modalities and currently leads online mantra meditation courses, international retreats, women's circles, and full/new moon gatherings.

Her jewelry line, Noelani Hawaii, combines intentional and healing crystals and natural materials to inspire women to feel beautiful, expressive, and empowered around the globe. Find Noelani's jewelry and retreats, events, and music online at NoelaniHawaii.com.

Flowing like the Honu

I have had so many amazing experiences surfing. I usually stick to my favorite surf breaks near my home. Every single time I play in the ocean, I see honu (the Hawaiian word for turtle). Turtles are completely in the flow. If you watch them swimming, they move really slowly, really fluidly, as if every stroke is a meditation. They have great breath practice (they can hold their breath for up to several hours), and they can also move swiftly when threatened. One of my favorite surfing memories happened at my favorite break, Ehukai sandbar. It was a beautiful spring day, and the waves were ideal for me, nice and small (two feet Hawaiian). I had been catching the inside waves because the outside was more crowded, and there was a long pause between sets. All of a sudden I saw a honu surface outside of everyone. I decided to swim out to it to

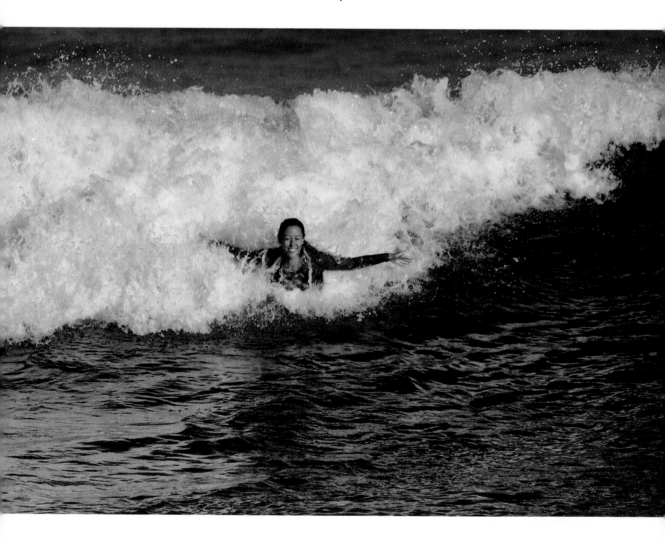

say aloha (I believe they are my aumakua, my Hawaiian spirit animal), and we glided underwater together for a moment before it swam off on its own. I came up for air, and there was a beautiful wave coming right for me. It peaked right where I was, and I swam for it and caught it all the way from the outside to the shoreline. I felt so euphoric sliding down the face of the wave, pressing my side body into the wave to hold my line. It was as if the turtle had guided me to the wave, showing me where to be in order to catch the set wave. Perhaps they're my ancestors, leading me to the perfect waves.

Having grown up as a competitive swimmer, I am much more comfortable being immersed in the water rather than being on top of a board. There are so many variables to consider while surfing—the current, the wind, positioning, being cautious of other surfers, making sure my swimsuit doesn't fall off, to name a few. Personally, bodysurfing is my favorite mode of wave riding. It allows me to be completely in the flow state, where I am fully present, as in meditation. The act of arriving at the water's edge is a ceremony for me, just like when I step onto my yoga mat. I set an intention, and I ask for safety, protection, and guidance from the spirit. Entering the womb of the earth, the place of mystery, depth, and the unknown of the powerful ocean, is a beautiful journey each time. I am humbled by the ocean, which is powerful enough to support life, but also able to take lives. Living on the North Shore of Oahu, we commonly experience tragic surf-related deaths, so honoring the force of nature is vital for my practice. In Hawaiian mythology, Kanaloa, the god of the ocean, is known for being unconquerable and immovable and represents the center of the universe within oneself.

Holding Your Breath under the Wave

I feel the glide of water along my skin and experience the pleasure of diving beneath the waves, eyes wide open, holding my breath, watching the white water of clouds roll over me, and I wait to surface again. I enjoy the challenge of finding the calm below the storm, the peace beneath the action above. There is a deep silence beneath the rumbling action on the surface, which for me is like a metaphor for life . . . being able to find the sweet spot when everything else is in constant motion or chaotic. I experience a lightness and sense of peace that for me is similar to orgasm. It's as if time stands still, and there's no sound, and I'm weightless. And then I come up for air and take in a deep gasp, as I've survived yet another deep dive into the unknown.

I swim to discover the right position to line up with the peak or shoulder of the wave and arrive in the place where it will pitch my body forward with the momentum of the water . . . so I can glide along the face of the wave, my body half in the water and half out. Like yoga, surfing keeps drawing me back to it. It's like I am always learning yet always humbled by the mystery, the growth, the challenge. It's similar when I get barreled: it's like I'm moving forward but I'm in a time warp; there's a void and the mystery of the portal. I think that's why guys love getting barreled so much, it's like being back in the womb, and the mystery of arriving on the other side keeps them wanting more.

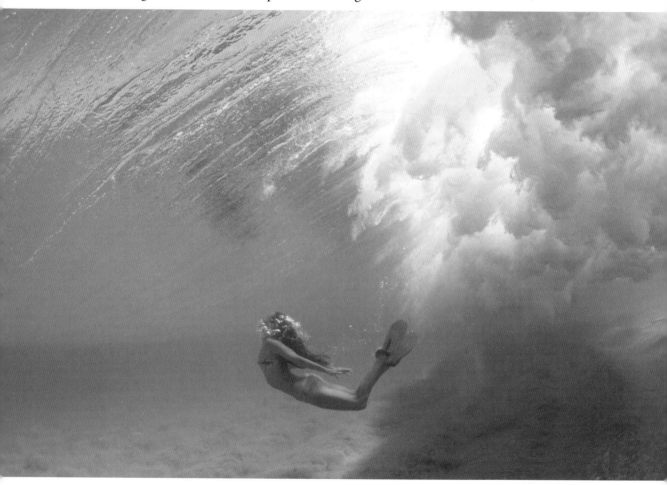

Noelani's Yoga for Surfing Practice

Here are a few of my favorite poses (asanas) that allow me to prepare for the day, as well as for surfing. The spine is the home of our central nervous system, so maintaining the proper structure and alignment of the spine is very important for overall health and wellness. These postures focus a lot on the spine, while also incorporating other features.

1. Lunge

Step one foot forward, bend your front knee to 90 degrees, keep your back leg slightly bent, and tuck your back toes. Feel your feet connected to the earth and engage your glutes and quads. Reach your arms down by your sides and clasp hands behind you. Draw your shoulders back and open the front of the chest. Breathe into your heart. Gaze up toward the sky if it feels OK for your neck, and feel the power emanating from your heart space. Take 5 breaths here. Repeat on the other leg.

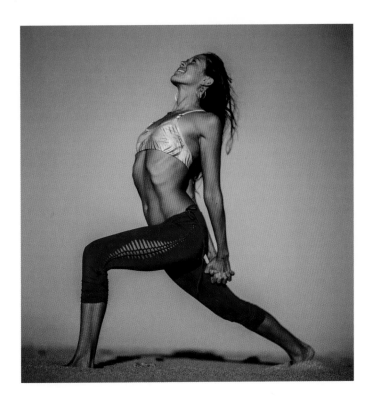

2. Seated Twist

Sit with legs extended in front of you, feet flexed. Place the left foot on the outside of the right knee or thigh. Reach both arms straight overhead, then twist to the left and wrap the right elbow around the knee, placing the left hand on the ground. Draw the shoulders back in their sockets and twist from the lower spine all the way into the head and neck. Inhale as you unwind slightly, and twist a little deeper on the exhale. Take 5 breaths here. Repeat on the other side.

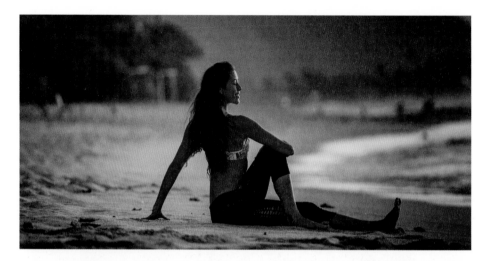

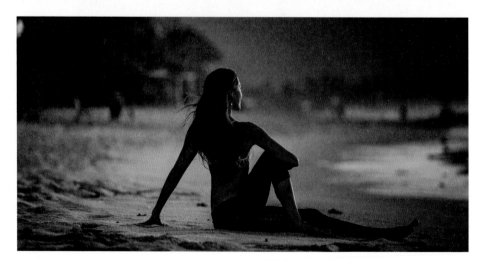

3. Seated Forward Fold

Extend both legs straight in front of you and flex your feet. Feel your sit bones grounded on the earth. Reach both arms up overhead and extend the arms forward as you fold. (If you have tight hamstrings, you can bend your knees.) The goal isn't necessarily to reach your feet at first; that will happen eventually as you gain flexibility. Avoid curving the lower spine, but rather hinge from the hips to create length through the back of the body. You can place your hands on your thighs, shins, feet, or whatever is accessible in the moment. Breathe in as you extend the spine, and exhale as you fold in. Take 5 breaths here.

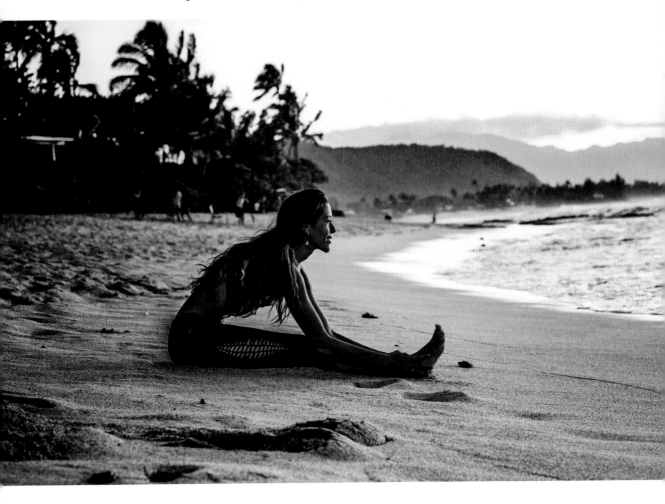

4. Camel

Kneel with your knees hip-distance apart. Place your hands on your lower back as if you were sliding your hands into your back pockets. Draw your shoulders into their sockets, away from the front of the chest, as you take a deep breath in and gently drop the head back. If this feels comfortable, stay here. If you'd like more of a stretch, you can place one hand at a time onto your ankles behind you to open

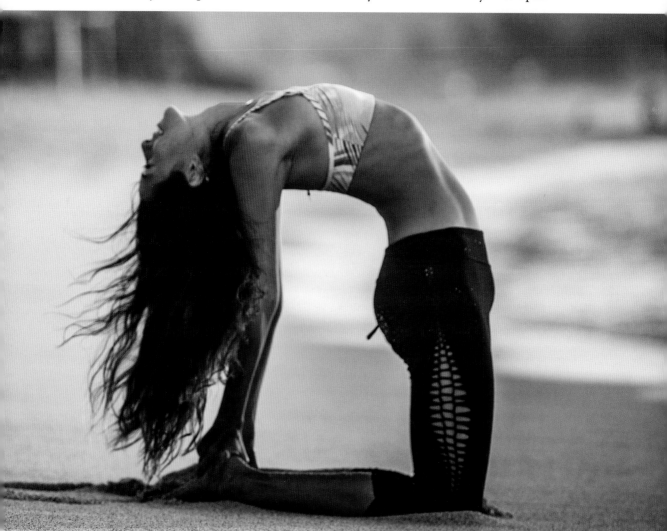

up the spine and the hips. Take 5 breaths in either variation. To come up from full camel, inhale slowly as you place your hands on the lower back and rise up. Be sure to take a counter pose such as child's pose, since this is an extreme heart opener.

Option: Instead of placing both hands on your ankles, extend one hand straight behind your head as shown in the photo here.

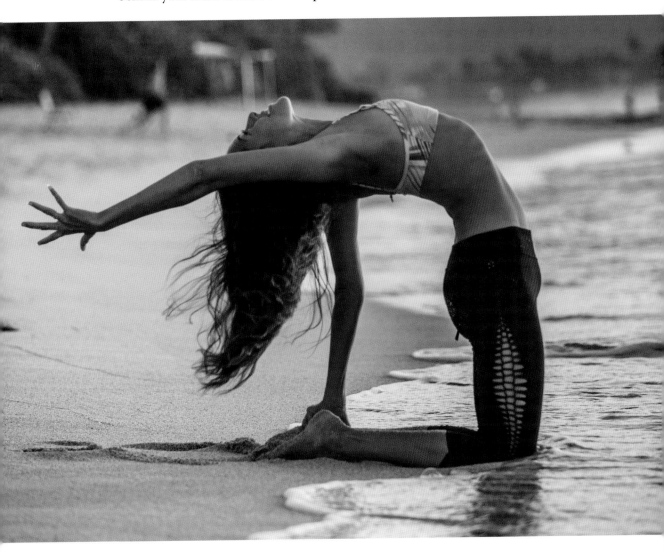

5. Lokah Samastah Mantra

Mantra: Lokah Samastah Sukhino Bhavantu

This mantra means: "May all beings everywhere be happy and free." Mantras are ancient chants/prayers that have been said for thousands of years, and this one comes from Sanskrit, which is one of the oldest languages on planet Earth and is said to have origins in the stars. This mantra can be sung or chanted at the beginning or end of a yoga practice to shift your vibration into one of intention and awakening. Chanting mantras is a way to activate the throat chakra (our center of truth and expression), and is a form of sound healing to bring conscious alignment to the cellular structure within the body.

Sit in a comfortable position; hands can be at heart center in anjali mudra or on the knees in gyan mudra. If you're a beginner, try chanting for 3 minutes to feel the vibratory effects of the words. (It's okay if you don't pronounce it exactly right; it's more about the essence and intention. If you do want to learn correct pronunciation, check out my song version here: noelanilove.bandcamp.com/track/lokah-samastah).

Eventually, as you get more comfortable with your voice and the mantra, chant for as long as you like. You may also choose to chant this mantra internally throughout your day to bring more peace to your own body and mind, as well as the world.

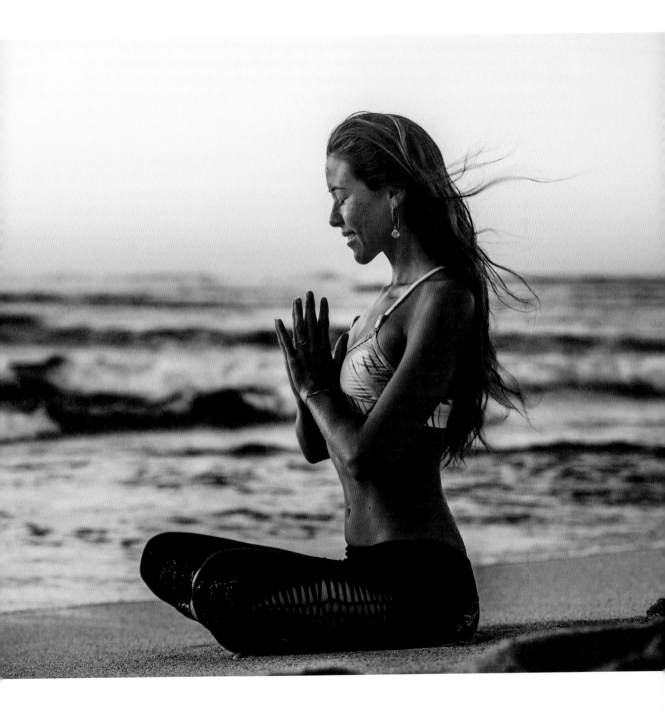

6. Rock Running

This is a Hawaiian practice for strength and breath training. You always want to practice this with a partner for safety reasons, as you may feel light-headed from lack of oxygen. You can practice this in depths of 7 feet or more. Beginners should stick to less than 10 feet, and as you progress, you can move to deeper water.

Find a rock that you can lift, but heavy enough to keep you weighted down for running on the sand bottom. Dive down, pressurizing your ears by holding your nose and blowing out your ears (or without plugging your nose if you're able to). Scoop up the rock and hold it in your hands or arms, however is comfortable for you. Your partner will then dive down and grab onto your shoulders for extra resistance as you run underwater. When you feel you are ready to come up for air, drop the rock (watch your feet!) and press up to the surface. Breathe and relax for at least a minute before going down again. Take turns with your partner. I like to do this about 5–10 times, but it depends on your breath-holding ability and your level of comfort underwater. Enjoy the relief of breathing in when you surface, and feel the burn in your legs.

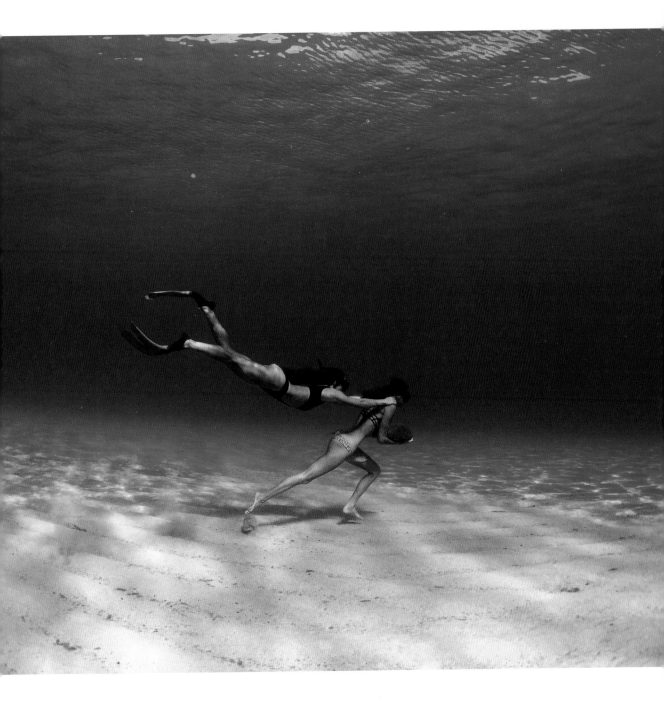

FalconGuides Interview: Get to Know Noelani Love

Q. Who or what brought you into yoga to begin with? How did you get started and what got you hooked?

A. Yoga and surfing are two of my dearest friends. They bring me great joy and peace and help me fall more in love with life. I'm able to laugh at myself through these practices, and, like true friends, they support my journey unconditionally. Yoga and surfing are some of my greatest teachers in life; the more I learn, the less I know, and the more eager I am to learn more. I thrive when I'm able to play in the ocean. I also work really hard, so I need yoga to stretch my body, as well as create more strength and integrity in my muscles. Plus, for true ocean lovers, when the waves aren't good, yoga is a great alternative to find the flow state.

For me, it's about finding a flow with my body. Being able to move fluidly with my breath is key to survival of my spirit. Being present in the moment is challenging with our overstimulated culture, so when I can be in complete flow, it helps me think more clearly, connect better with humans, and define who I am.

Q. What about surfing? How did that happen? Who, what, when, where, and why did you start and what has that journey been like?

A. I grew up dreaming about being a surfer girl. My surfing adventure began on the shores of Waikiki as a child. I was born and raised in Charlotte, North Carolina, to a Hawaiian mother and a southern gentleman father. I swam on a summer league swim team, and when the season was over, my mother would take the children (my older brother, younger sister, and I) to Hawaii to visit our grandparents for the last month of summer vacation. My parents and grandparents weren't really into surfing, but they loved being at the beach and being in the ocean, and they encouraged us to love being in the water, whether it was the pool or the ocean. I would play in the shore break with my siblings and cousins, getting tumbled in the sand, as my mom would say, "in the washing machine." I eventually began to venture out farther with a bodyboard, and then took my first surf lesson with my brother in Waikiki as a teenager. That was how we spent our summers, playing in the waves all day every day, and snorkeling to view the wildlife when there were no waves.

Q. Can you describe your first or most transcendent experience with yoga? Anything that made you experience the flow state we are talking about in this book?

A. I had my first cathartic experience during a kundalini yoga class where we were invited to sing a mantra (sacred yogic chant) during a kriya (series of posture, breath, and sound). My son's father and I had recently divorced, and I had been so busy working on jewelry production and sales and taking care of my child that I hadn't allowed myself to process the feelings of the breakup. I simply didn't have the time and space to do so. All of a sudden, as I was seated on the floor with my legs spread into a V for wide-legged side bends, singing this unfamiliar series of foreign words, I started bawling. I wasn't sure what was happening, but it felt good. I felt freedom and release. I felt relieved. I later realized I had been holding on to feelings of hurt, shame, grief, pain, regret, and sadness that I had never allowed to move through me. I knew I needed more of this healing in my life. I eventually signed up for my first yoga teacher training, a kundalini training with my teacher Gurmukh in India. She taught me about kriyas, breath, mudras, and, most of all, trust in the divine. I was going through a very challenging transition in my business during this time. I sought counsel from Gurmukh, and her simple response was: "Noelani, keep playing your ukulele." I went home to Hawaii to open a new yoga studio/retail boutique and record my first album, a full collection of ancient Hawaiian, Sufi, Sanskrit, and yoga traditions. My intention with the album is to encourage people to sing along to the sacred chants (which are repetitive and easy to learn, as well as having been sung for thousands of years as prayers to lift our spirits) and to find their own empowered voices to create change on our planet. When we can tune in to the healing power of our own voices, I feel that we can create ripples of healing around the world.

Q. What about surfing? Was there an experience that stands out more than the rest, and can you describe it in words? Where were you?

A. A few places that I've traveled to on earth have allowed me to connect to the energy of flow state that I feel when I'm practicing yoga, surfing, and singing. The culture of the tropics resonates with my spirit. When I studied abroad in Costa Rica during my college years, I was so inspired and I reconnected with my love of surfing and dance. I also have a strong connection to Hawaii obviously, the place of my ancestors. The islands are truly magical. Bali is also a power point for me, as it is a magnetic vortex of consciousness, stimulating growth and creativity for me, and I feel that the magma movement within these volcanic islands can be felt and is very supportive of my own creative process. As the islands birth, so shall I . . . more in the practice of singing/songwriting/artistic creativity and embodied movement. I feel the mana (life force in the Hawaiian language) strongly from the earth in these places, and I enjoy allowing myself to be a channel of energy flowing.

Q. Where and how did you start out in yoga? What was your first introduction to the practice and how do you suggest people start if they are considering getting into yoga? What is your favorite style to practice? Do you teach yoga? If so, what style?

A. I used to hate yoga. The beginning of my relationship with yoga is a funny one. I remember one day at the beach in Waikiki, around the age of eleven, hearing the word *yoga* in conversation and asking my mom what it was. She showed me a side plank pose, and I thought it was weird. Later, as a nineteen-year-old college student in Virginia, I attended a few yoga classes with friends, and I remember being frustrated that our teacher was teaching us how to breathe. I found myself comparing my body to my friend, who could fold her head down to her knee.

I came to the realization (as probably everyone succumbs to at some point during their yogic path) that I wasn't "good at yoga," so I quit. I had way more important things to do at the time, like go to frat parties and smoke weed with my friends. I thought yoga was silly, and I decided I wouldn't go back again.

Lesson #1 in yoga: no comparing. Everyone has a different body and a different story, and we all arrive at different places at different times. That is why yoga is called a "practice." The more you do it, the better you get.

I didn't venture back to the wonderful world of yoga until the age of twenty-three, living in Hawaii as a recent college graduate. I had just starting my jewelry business and was modeling, go-go dancing, and doing alcohol promotions on the side for extra money. My brother (who also lived in Hawaii) would take me surfing in Waikiki at some popular spots, and although determined and excited to surf, I had a hard time shortboarding with the crowds and the fast waves that he loved and always took me to. After a year of being deeply embedded in the nightlife scene of Honolulu on the south shore of the island of Oahu, I decided to move to the North Shore, which is the home of some of the best waves in the world. I wanted to have easier access to clean water, good waves with less crowds, and a simpler life than that of living in the big city of Honolulu. After moving to the North Shore of Oahu, I started playing around with bodyboarding and bodysurfing because having a board in the big waves seemed dangerous to me and I felt like a danger to the other surfers around me. Plus, growing up as a competitive swimmer, I am much more comfortable being immersed in the water rather than on top of a board. I enjoyed having a less dangerous option than a fiberglass board with sharp fins, and the easy commitment of a boogie or just my body.

My partner at the time and I soon found out I was pregnant, and I started to recognize that I wanted to take better care of my body for the health of my growing baby. One day, while treating myself to lunch at a newly discovered local vegetarian cafe called Paradise Found near my new North Shore home, I saw a sign for "prenatal yoga." I decided that I wanted to make friends with other pregnant women so that we could support each other in this new chapter of life. (Most of my party friends were definitely not in the phase of becoming moms.)

I checked out the class, and I immediately loved the energy of Mara, our teacher. I enjoyed taking time out of my busy work schedule to be instructed and not have to think about all the "things on the to-do list." I enjoyed how she instructed us to move with our breath and move our bodies in ways that I hadn't allowed myself to do before without shame. She guided us though hip circles, stretches, and power poses for our changing bodies and growing babies. Mara invited us to place our hands over our wombs during class, say hello to our babies, and feel the energy of the sacred being growing inside of each of us. That class changed my life. Simply taking seventy-five minutes to connect with my body and breath while growing a baby activated a deeply intuitive sense of motherhood within me that I didn't know existed. It inspired and prepared me for the home birth I would eventually have with my son.

Yoga classes kept drawing me back. I was beginning to be more in tune with my body and felt strong, empowered, and more aware of how I moved. After an amazing home birth experience with my beautiful baby boy, I began attending mom and baby yoga, so that I could connect and relate with other moms who also had milk squirting out of their breasts and spent their days changing diapers. Once my son was old enough to leave with a sitter, I began going to yoga classes with one of my surfer friends, Kendyl, at a recreation center nearby. My favorite thing about this class was that I could be alone on my mat. Nobody needed me. There was no need for me to communicate to anyone. Just me, my body, my breath, my heart, and my mind in my space. After a full day of breastfeeding, a sleepless night, and simply trying to get through the day with 1) a healthy meal, 2) a shower, and 3) maybe having time to comb my hair . . . yoga was heaven. As a new mother, this hour of focus with my breath and body was extremely healing for my exhausted mind and body. I began attending more and more classes with different teachers of different styles. I was starting to fall in love with yoga!

I know that starting a yoga practice can be intimidating. Remember, I quit after just a few classes because my friend could fold her head down to her knee and I couldn't! If you're curious or interested in starting a yoga practice, I believe that the key is to try different types of yoga, and try different teachers. I know a lot of people who say they went to one class and didn't like it, so they never tried it again. There are a multitude of styles and a large variety of teachers who teach in different ways. Every teacher will put their own spin on the teachings, as they have each gone through different life experiences. For example, I've been trained in kundalini yoga, vinyasa flow, and mantra yoga, as well as prenatal yoga and children's yoga. I incorporate all these styles into my personal practice and teachings, because that's what I know and understand, and it works with my lifestyle as a woman and as a mom. I appreciate adding in humor and fun as well as fluidity and breath work and mantra into my practice, because I value the teachings and understand that all these modalities have very important lessons to share. I think finding a teacher that you can resonate with and appreciate will help you tremendously in building a solid foundation of a practice.

The goal isn't to be the "best yogi" or the "best surfer," but rather to be in the present with your body, heart, and mind. I think anyone at any level can access a feeling of flow state in yoga or surfing. I believe this experience is easily accessible as long as you have breath awareness. I find myself in the flow state in moments of cooking, free diving, making love, and even when I was in the throes of labor with my son.

Three tips:

1. Breathe.
2. Have fun.
3. Don't judge or compare yourself to others.

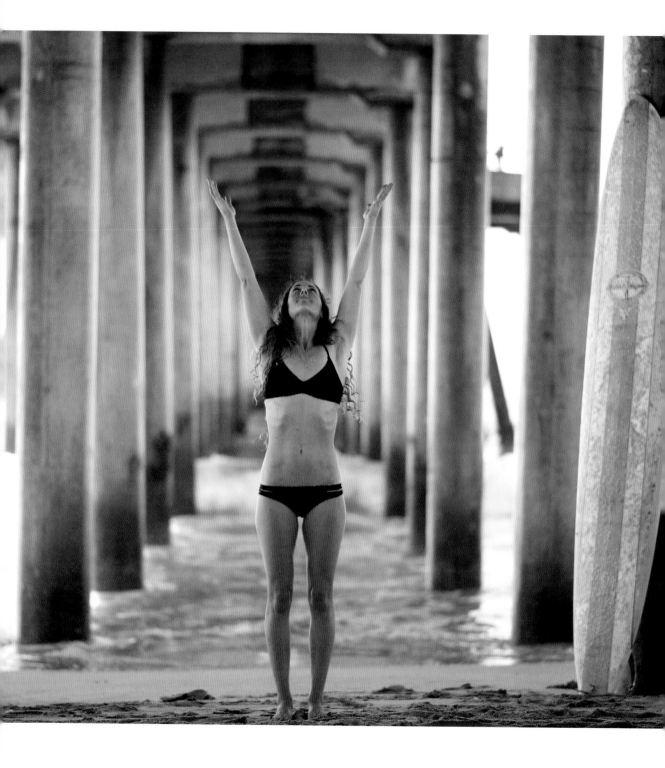

GURU YOGA FOR SURFERS

Jessi Moon

Anytime you are feeling anything other than happiness and peace it is only serving as a reminder to get back in touch with yourself.

—*Sai Steven S. Sadleir*

About Jessi

Jessi Moon shares her wisdom of yoga, meditation, and mindfulness in Orange County, California, where she visits homes for private lessons and counsels children to heal their behavior problems by empowering them with tools to feel peace and happiness. She is a public speaker and teacher on Conscious Parenting and holds Mindfulness Teacher trainings and retreats with her guru. To join her in a class with her guru, visit SelfAwareness.com and become a member to join the weekly teleconferenced classes. Jessi is a senior teacher at the Self Awareness Institute, an organization dedicated to bringing light and love into the world through every aspect of life. Her website is LetsEnlightenTogether.com.

As you keep practicing meditation, you will get a lot of happiness and bliss. The kind of happiness you get in meditation does not exist anywhere on this earth. All the kinds of happiness you experience outside are nothing compared to the happiness you get when you meditate.

—*Sri Sri Sri Shivabalayogi Maharaj*

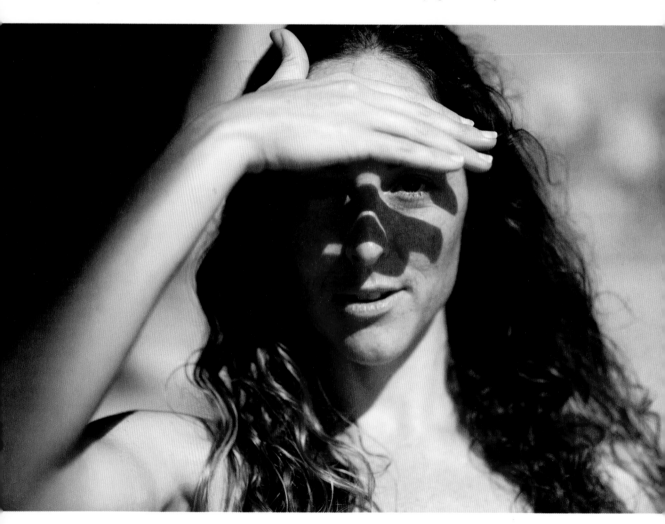

Jessi's Yoga for Surfing Practice

The practice that I'd like to share with you is a third eye kundalini shaktipat meditation. This is the meditation my guruji gave to me; it brings me deep, elated states of blissfulness and into samadhi ("putting together"), to become one with God or consciousness. It is what yoga is all about and what sets a basic yoga practice apart from a mind-blowing, blissful, advanced yoga practice.

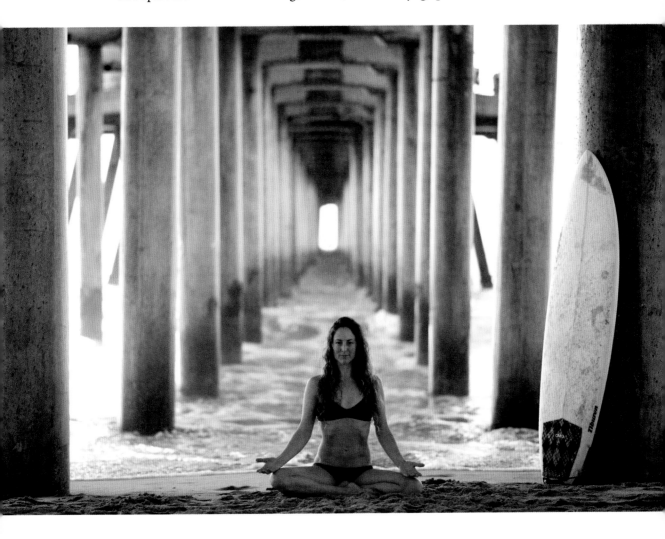

After you practice your yoga postures, breathing exercises, mantras, eye gazing, or whatever other techniques you like to practice, do this meditation: Sit up straight, like a sitting yogi. You don't have to sit on the ground; you just need to have a straight spine with shoulders rolled back and be as comfortable as possible. Use pillows to prop yourself up if that feels good. But make sure to have a straight spine. Then close your eyes, roll them up to the point between the eyebrows, and gently focus your attention there. Gaze into the black screen of your mind here and focus on the light at this point.

It will take a bit of time to open your third eye. If you can find a guru in your area, the guru can help you to open your third eye and awaken your kundalini for you. This is how it was done for me. But we can connect psychically, too, and you're welcome to join our online classes at the Self Awareness Institute to really get it. Basically you simply focus on this point and imagine your breath moving in and out through this point as if white light were moving in and out of your forehead. Imagine you're under a waterfall of light, and with each exhale you let go of all your thoughts and imagine them streaming out through this point, and with every inhale you breathe in that waterfall of loving light in through the point between your eyebrows.

With practice, you will begin entering into deeper and deeper states that will bring you deeper and deeper peace, love, and clarity. I recommend working with a trained teacher. Like anything you learn in life, if you find a good teacher who is sincere in their practice and knowledge, and one who is also acknowledged in a lineage, then you will be more adept at attaining yoga (self-realization or enlightenment).

The other tool I can give you is the S.T.O.P. tool. This is a mindfulness tool to help you stay conscious. Anytime you feel out of flow you Stop, Take a deep breath, Observe yourself and the situation (step out of your head), and gain Perspective on peace and love by asking, "What can I do in the moment to create more peace and love?" Then allow inspiration to flow through you to resolve your problem! Anytime you do something that creates more peace and love, it is the right thing to do. It is also important to understand that anything you do that creates more suffering and chaos, even if you feel it is the "right" thing to do, is the wrong thing to do. So we have to have the humility of mind to be able to S.T.O.P. ourselves, humble the mind, and remember that love is the way. It's not about being right; it's about love.

Jessi's Favorite Yoga for Surfing Poses

1. Mountain Pose

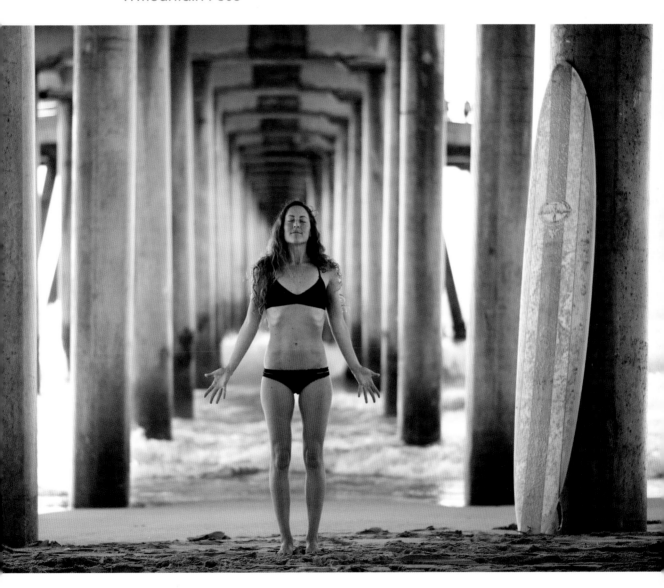

2. Upward-Facing Dog

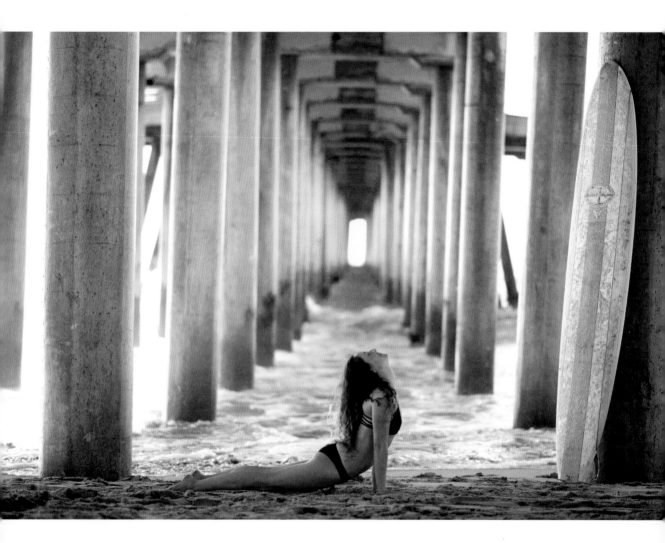

3. Chaturanga

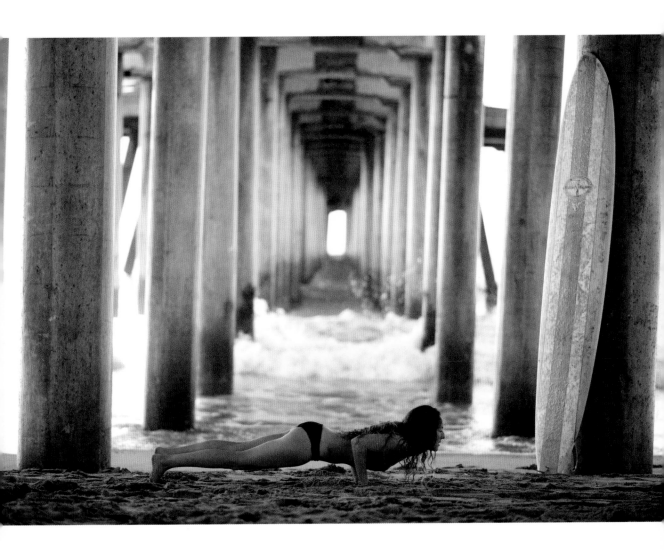

4. Side Angle Pose

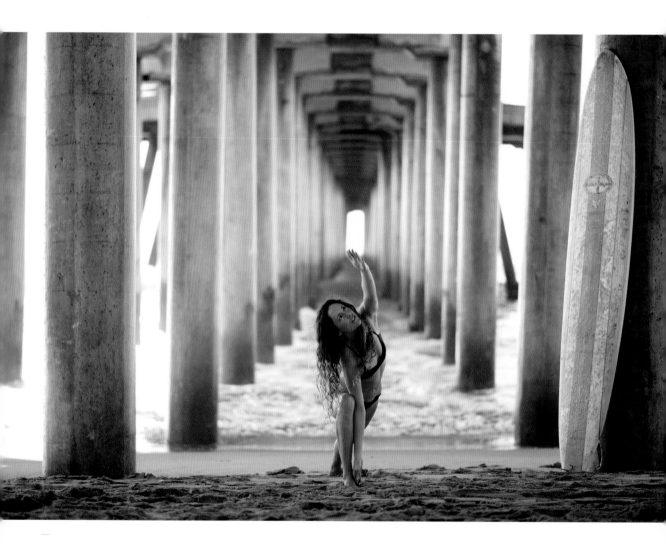

5. Headstand

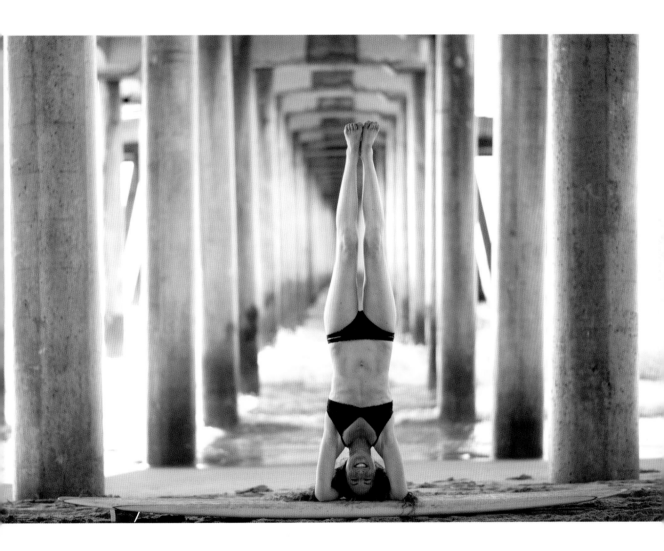

Jessi's Tips to Help You Get More from Life

> Once you realize that the world is your own projection, you are free of it.
>
> —*Nisargadatta Maharaj*

I recommend people meditate every day for an hour. When you reach this phase, your life is a lot better and you live more clearly and in a powerful loving flow. Learning to control the mind and enter into higher states of consciousness (Sat Chit Ananda) is the key to a wonderful, blissful life.

Make sure you play every day, whether that means surfing or dancing in your room. Surf whenever you can if you're lucky enough to live near the beach and find windows in your workday to paddle out. It's all about priorities. Surfing for me is a priority; if I don't surf, I'm not as happy as I could be. It's important to play in God's kingdom. It's like worship to the divine to feel so immersed with God. Surfing is similar to living life and navigating the waves of energy all around us every day. Sometimes you jump on and ride in the flow, following every curve so perfectly, and sometimes you completely wipe out and get brutally beaten. I feel like I'm playing with God when I surf, riding His every move, I feel His exaltation and power.

I like to experience life to its fullest. I didn't have any drugs during childbirth, not because it didn't hurt, but because I wanted to feel what it was to be a woman. I want to *feel* life. Life is an experience, and it's beautiful and magical. We've been evolving for millions of years . . . and here we are. Yoga and meditation are becoming mainstream, and those that practice with sincerity are like super-beings. No matter what you do in life, the practice of yoga, including the practice of meditation, will bring you greater happiness, peace, and wisdom. Yoga teaches you to be in the flow, riding waves everywhere you go. Let's surf our way through this universe and ride these waves of energy all around us.

It's all guiding you to your best self, where you can serve humanity and make a difference in the world. We all have unique gifts and are here to bring a higher awareness and love into the world, not through someone else's idea, but through your own direct realization of higher truths and higher love. You have been chosen, like me. Some of you may already know this, but for those who don't, may I be the one to invite you into your true awakened self! Alakh Niranjan! May the in-dwelling spirit within you awaken! It's the best thing that will ever happen to you, and you will no longer care so much about trivial problems in your life. You will see a greater purpose and connect with others on a higher plane—similar to how Dashama and I have found each other. We've never met in person; our spirits just connected to bring this awareness to you. The energy within us *is* us. You are a part of it, too.

> The three main ways that man wastes his energy are Greed, Anger and Worry.
>
> —*Yogiraj Vethathiri Maharishi*

The kingdom of heaven is right here on earth. This is what Jesus said in the gospel of Thomas in some of the earliest writings we have on Jesus's words, He said, "For the Kingdom of Heaven is spread out before man, yet he sees it not, for those that have eyes let them see." My guruji taught me the truths that all great avatars spoke about. We have misinterpreted many of the spiritual leaders of our world and turned their teachings into false teachings that made authorities wealthy and superior. Buddha was a yogi, he had a guru, and he meditated under a bodhi tree until he enlightened. Jesus meditated and prayed for forty days and forty nights in the desert; my guru did his tapas in India where he sat for forty days and forty nights twenty-three hours per day under the guidance of his guru, Shiva Bala Yogi Maharaj, who also did tapas and began sitting at the young age of thirteen for twenty-three hours per day for eight years, then twelve hours per day for another twelve years, and basically sat his entire life in a transcended state to be a powerhouse of light for the world. All the great saints who lived on our planet meditated and taught to look within to find yourself or to find God.

Yoga is the science of self-realization or God realization. And it is available for anyone who wants to learn who they are and why they are here and how they can live in their highest happiness and peace with control over the mind. We're here to manifest heaven on earth, but our minds are what prevent us from bringing this love into the world. By learning to control the mind and understand ourselves better, we can balance our energy and generate more of our life force energy or spirit too, which is love! We are all here to bring light into the world, and the way to generate more light and love is through the practice of yoga.

Real yoga, though, includes meditation. The yoga postures are simply meant to clear the body of stress and open energy pathways for a deeper, more powerful meditation. The postures are the foundation to a good life and pain-free blissful meditation, and great surfing too! When your energy is clear and you touch upon every muscle, releasing its stress in your body, you have greater use and awareness of your body, which allows better balance on your board and in your life. Isn't it better to live without pain, excessive stress, and a frantic mind?

Bhakti (devotion) is a big part of yoga, too. To have a guru to show the way has been key for my development in my practice. Find a great teacher and listen. The guru is the one who holds the highest vibration, who emanates God's love, who has purified his body-mind vehicle to serve humanity, and who brings a powerful love into the world. I feel like one of the luckiest people in the world to have found such a beautiful guru to help guide me on my path. We are all being guided, we were meant to connect. I would love to continue supporting you on your journey in yoga, which means union with God in a nonreligious sense, or in other words, union of the body and mind with that which sustains, creates, and draws life back into itself—the beholder or sustainer of all that exists, Shiva. To the essence within you that is also within me I serve.

FalconGuides Interview: Get to Know Jessi Moon

Q. Who or what brought you into yoga to begin with? How did you get started and what got you hooked?

A. I first started practicing yoga when I was eighteen years old. I was just learning to surf that year too. My friend Jay, who was teaching me to surf, and I were eating at a health food store, and across the street was a yoga studio. So we decided to go try. I think we both did their free week of yoga. It was the Bikram-style hot yoga series. We were both hooked, and I ended up working at the studio a few hours a week in trade for yoga classes. This studio was the first studio that had the full Bikram hot yoga series but also had other styles of yoga, including a meditation class. Bikram actually tried to sue this studio for having other kinds of yoga practiced in their studio, but the studio ended up winning the case. I'm so grateful they won because if you go to an all-Bikram studio you never learn how to meditate, which is the whole purpose of yoga.

This studio is also where I met my guruji, Steven S. Sadleir, who also goes by SAI, a name given to him by the great avatar Sai Baba. It also stands for the Self Awareness Institute, which he founded in the 1980s in response to the encouragement of his root guru, Yogiraj Vethathiri Maharishi, a kundalini master from the Tamil lineage. Steven had a meditation class on Monday nights. It was the last class of the day, so after I checked everyone in, I would slip in to the class every Monday night. Sometimes the phone would ring, so I'd have to quietly get up and go answer it, but Steven was always supportive of me learning and saw my sincerity in wanting to learn more. I was fascinated in his class with what he said and my experiences with him.

This yoga studio was my sanctuary. I was eighteen years old just looking for my way in life after graduating from high school, wondering what I should study in college and what I wanted to do with my life. I would journal often, and the answers were always, I want to study who I am and what is life. I thought about studying philosophy in college, but it wasn't exactly what I was looking for. I didn't want to philosophize about life, I wanted to know it. What was that study? I wandered . . . so when I found yoga, or really when I found Steven, a master of yoga and meditation, I realized this was it. This was what I wanted to study, and it gave me a practice to look within to get the answers I sought.

Finding a master to learn from directly has been the key for me, and the most loving experience of my life. What makes a master is commitment, sincerity, and dedication. I've never seen any human being on this earth have more dedication, commitment, and reverence or love (bhakti) for God or spirit and serving humanity than Steven. Yoga is all about love. Find a teacher you love and who has a sincere heart, who has studied yoga, and preferably one who meditates daily. This is a yogi. Anyone claiming they are a guru or yoga teacher who does not practice meditation is a bogi, a false yogi, and we have many here in America. That's not to say they are not teaching something that is still good and helpful, like the yoga postures or breathing exercises, but it is important to know the difference. If you really want to study and learn yoga, you find a good teacher.

A guruji's ancient wisdom is sacred and has been passed down for thousands of years. We need more sincere students learning from true powerful lineages. I would never have known a fraction of what I do today, or have had the capability to find such elated states of bliss and clarity within me, without my guruji. Many Americans feel they can "get it on their own," and this is only the ego talking. The ego is the very thing the guru will smash out of you to purify you to attain enlightenment. The Bikram series helped heal my scoliosis and push energy though my body to open me up *and* I found a master in the studio, so I consider myself one of the luckiest yogini's in the world! But the divine is guiding you, too, and it's brought us together through these words, so you are a part of this lineage now, and I look forward to sharing more with you in spirit as spirit.

What hooked me into continuing to practice after that first free week of yoga was the feeling I got from the Bikram series and the idea that I could learn to master something new and heal my body, too. It was a true yoga studio; I met some of the nicest people in the world here, and there was true unconditional love. It was a fun time in my life.

Love is all that matters.

—*Sai Steven S. Sadleir*

Q. What about surfing? How did that happen? Who, what, when, where, and why did you start and what has that journey been like?

A. Surfing was something I always wanted to learn since I was a little girl. I was just always so small and skinny and the ocean was big and cold. It wasn't till I turned eighteen that I felt strong enough to take on the challenge to teach myself. My friend Jay took me to San Onofre State Beach in California, a place where it's like heaven on earth. The waves are mellow and it's a great place to learn. The people are supernice, and many families go here to enjoy the gentle rolling waves, sun, and breezy air. San Onofre is one of my favorite places to surf. It's a great place to learn to longboard. Longboarding is an easy way to learn to surf if you can find a beach with gentle, rolling waves like San O. So when Jay first took me to San Onofre to learn, he pushed me into my first few waves and I stood up right away. Once I got that feeling, I was like *wow*! After that it was just about getting my arms strong enough to paddle myself in, which didn't take too long.

I dedicated myself to surf every day. I figured even if I didn't catch a wave, at least I paddled around and was getting stronger and used to the ocean. The ocean is like a dance partner. You have to get to know it, how it moves; every day is different, it has so many moods. Some days it's calm and pretty and others it's stormy and raining. No matter what the ocean's mood was, I was out there! Sometimes all alone even! But on those days when I was alone, when it was raining and storming, I felt so alive! So close to God. The key to learning to surf is to surf. When you're learning, you have to go every day, or at least a few times a week to really get it. It's fun challenging yourself to learn to surf! It's a hard sport to learn! Anyone can do it, but it just takes dedication and maybe a loving friend to help show you your first few times (and it helps if they give you a board too!).

May the whole world live in happiness and peace.
—*Sai Steven S. Sadleir*

Q. Can you describe your first or most transcendent experience with yoga? Anything that made you experience the flow state we are talking about in this book?

A. My teacher Steven gives retreats every so often, and these retreats have been the most incredible experiences in my life. Steven is a master, so we are not just practicing yoga poses and breathing exercises. We meditate, a lot. He comes around and touches our third eye and send his shakti (life force energy) into our being so we can enter into transcendental planes of consciousness bliss. Having my third eye touched by Steven is like if an angel were to come and send a love powerful enough to blow your mind. We all have a spirit within us, but not everyone's spirit is awakened. When a guru touches your third eye, they help awaken your kundalini energy, which is the energy that runs up and down your spine. It is the energy that moves through the chakras, rotating in a clockwise direction up your spine, and there are exercises, breathing techniques, and other ways to help awaken it through the practice of yoga. But when you're working with a master who has had his kundalini awakened and soaring and has established himself so strongly in this energy, it becomes effortless in his presence to awaken your own. Steven simply transfers his shakti and you receive it. He has so much divine love that being around him brings you into samadhi effortlessly.

Samadhi is the goal in yoga; it is the state in meditation where *you* no longer exist. It is hard to explain, but it is where your individual consciousness merges with the total consciousness and you realize your true self. I've been so elated at these retreats, there's no way to describe the experience in words—only tears of joy, my mind blown and feeling so full of love and bliss. We are all able to reach elated states; yoga teaches us the way. If you are struggling in your life, in your yoga practice, or in surfing, it is simply because you have to let go of needing anything to be different. The guru is within me and within you; it's not just in the physical guru like guruji Steven. The physical guru like Steven is simply an enlightened being who has practiced and perfected his consciousness to abide in this higher, elated state. So being around a master of yoga will influence you to also look within, and will help guide you like a father to connect with the guru within you. The guru is spirit itself, and spirit expressed is love. Love is the teacher. and the physical guru is really a master of love and sharing love and light. May we all become masters of connecting to this love and light within us, and share that love with everyone we see everywhere we go all the time every day.

Q. What about surfing? Was there an experience that stands out more than the rest, and can you describe it in words? Where were you?

A. I've had so many incredible experiences surfing, I especially love big waves, but I have to be careful because I have dislocated my shoulder a few times. One time I dislocated it after pulling out of a huge set wave. The wave flung me up in the air as I pulled out to get out of it before it walled up and I got smashed, but I barely made it out. And when I was pulling up the face, it was breaking down, so I raced up and out as fast as I could. It launched me really high, and when I came down, the water just pushed my arm out of the socket. I have a weak shoulder from a snowboard accident, and it's also genetic. My dad dislocates his shoulder sometimes, too. I was so scared when I dislocated it out in the ocean on a big wave day though. I screamed my head off in pain and fear of dying from the next big wave crashing on me. I was at the Huntington Beach pier, my home spot, and all the guys paddled over to help. There was a wave coming, so they were going to just put me on my board and send me in. I knew I wasn't going to be able to stay on the board holding on with only one arm and in excruciating pain, so I frantically repeated, "Please don't leave me, please don't leave me, I'm going to fall off, I can't do it. Please don't leave me!" And at the last minute, a young surfer guy jumped on top of me, grabbed me and my board, and rode me in safely. He saved my life; I could have drowned. My arm went back into the socket as I relaxed it while we were riding in. This was a pretty intense experience, but it made me feel really good knowing the guys out there are strong loving men. I usually surf alone. I make friends wherever I go and enjoy being in the moment with whomever I may be near. But I love being alone.

To me surfing is like living in heaven, riding God's waves in his kingdom playing as life was meant to be lived.

Q. Are there specific places on earth where you feel most connected to this energy or flow state of consciousness, whether you are practicing yoga, surfing, both, or just being?

A. I feel connected wherever I go. You don't need to be anywhere in particular to be connected. It's a state we seek in yoga, not a place, but the beach is definitely a place that can bring me back into the flow. Being in nature is important for all of us. If I'm in a funk, feeling stuck, and so forth, there are three go-tos for me: meditation, yoga, and surfing. When you combine all three and add in my guru to the mix. WOW. I got my guru Steven surfing awhile back, and he's been doing it ever since now. We like to go to San Onofre State Beach together. We practice some yoga postures on the beach, go out for a little surf, come back in, then do a meditation on the berm of the beach. Those are my most cherished days. So the order is yoga (stretch), surf (play), meditate (commune with the divine), then go eat tacos. This is my favorite sequence to reset my entire being to humming in the glory of life.

Q. Can you name your favorite surf break and where that is? What about for new surfers, is there a best place to learn in your opinion? Did you start with lessons or just go out and take the waves on? Is your family into surfing or were you a pioneer in your family?

A. My favorite surf break is probably Church. It's in front of the marine base in San Clemente, so it's a bit of a trek to get there, but it's by far the best wave around. It's a point break, so it peels and creates a long right. I've had some amazing days at Church. I love that usually there's not a lot of people out, since it is harder to get to.

My other favorite spot is the Huntington Beach pier, my home spot. My dad moved to Huntington when he was younger because of this wave. He also used to drive down to Trestles, which is where Church and Lowers is, and get chased off the marine base. Back then they didn't want surfers out in front of the marine base. They used to sneak out and ride the waves and then run from the marines! (I have the coolest dad.) I dislocated my shoulder once at Church, so I was really far from my car and had to walk up to the marine base and ask for help. One of the marines asked, "Do you have permission to be on the base?" In a pompous tone, I looked at him angrily and said, "My shoulder dislocated and I need help!" They brought an ambulance on the base to take me to the hospital.

My third favorite spot is Newport. I love to shortboard, too; it's my new thing. The waves in Newport are really fast and they break *hard*, so I have to be careful with my shoulder. Newport is right below my house now. Blackies is a break at the Newport Beach pier that I like to take my son to. He loves to bodysurf, and it's a great spot for kids to learn.

I have to mention San Onofre too. Old Mans, too. I have so many spots, I honestly don't have a favorite. Old Mans is good when I just want to be crazy and hang out with friends. I go longboarding here. I'm the kind of surfer that surfs on all boards and all breaks. I truly love the ocean and surfing waves—snorkeling and diving too. I love to bodysurf with my son, or we use boogie boards—we have these mini boogies that are fun and get you right in the pocket. I'm like a mermaid. I love dolphins too. On Mother's Day last year I decided I wanted to surf first thing that morning and see some dolphins. My son and I went down to Newport, I paddled out, and two dolphins swam directly up to me and right under me! I had actually paddled out and sat for a minute looking around with the intention of seeing them, and a few minutes later there they were! It was almost like they had heard my call. The ocean is a magical place, and the creatures that live in the sea are incredibly intelligent. They can feel you and are very psychic creatures. They love to play. I always paddle up to them when I see them, and sometimes they surf with us too!

Just as there is diversity in all things, I recommend learning all types of surfing. Just get out and play in the sea! Sometimes I just go for a dip and jump up and down and throw myself around on the shore. My son and I love to do this. We hold hands and jump around bodysurfing, roll up on the beach, throw sand at each other, run around, maybe do some handstands or other yoga poses, make a drip castle, then go jump around like a baby seal in the waves again. My son loves to jump on my back when I catch a wave. The ocean is a gift from God.

Q. Where and how did you start out in yoga? What was your first introduction to the practice and how do you suggest people start if they are considering getting into yoga? What is your favorite style to practice? Do you teach yoga? If so, what style?

A. I first started out in yoga as a teenager, as I mentioned earlier. I was eighteen years old and worked the front desk at a studio to get free yoga classes. It was Bikram-style yoga that I learned first, which was perfect for my young body that needed healing and transformation. Now, similar to my approach to surfing, I practice all styles of yoga. All yoga is good—there is not one style that is better than another. Sometimes you need different styles for the different moods and phases in your life. It's all about listening to the satguru (inner teacher); listen to your body and follow what serves you best in the moment. Developing this self-awareness is something we attain in the yoga practice. Some days you will feel more like taking a restorative yoga class, and other days you may feel like taking a Bikram hot yoga class. They all serve you. If you listen to your body, it will tell you what it needs. A good way to do this if you are unsure what would best serve you is to ask. Simply ask in your mind in a meditative state: "What can I do in this moment to feel better? What practice or series would best serve me? Should I go surfing?" And then just listen. Sometimes the answer is to do your yoga on the beach, then surf, then meditate on the berm! Sometimes the answer is stay home, take a bath, and do some restorative poses on the floor and with your swing. (I have a yoga swing in my room that I love so much.) It's all about honoring your body and learning to bring yourself into elated states of pure mind and pristine energy. Meditating every day will help you calm your mind and make you more insightful as to how to better guide yourself through life.

I am a yoga teacher, but my emphasis is on meditation and self-awareness or mindfulness. I use the postures with my clients for healing and clearing out the body, but it is not the focus of what I teach. The focus is on love—being there for somebody, supporting them through their life experiences, and giving them the tools to live a happier and more powerful life. I work with a lot of children and am known as kind of a child whisperer. If a child is troubled, many times having a few sessions with me will give them what they need. I leave them with tools and a higher awareness on how to deal with their life better so they don't experience anxiety and so forth. Children are very open, and they don't always make the best students, but neither do adults. I feel if I can reach children, support them while they're young, then as they grow they will remember and will continue to grow their awareness and their practice and become more and more powerful. We need more powerful beings on our planet to help change it. We need more people awakening and making a difference in the world. Children are the future, and many are troubled due to troubled parents and other adults around them. So we need to help people and kids learn yoga, learn how to meditate, learn how to become more self-aware or mindful so we can end unnecessary suffering. You are an incarnation of light and love; if you're not living in the love of your underlying essence, you need to practice yoga! Spread the word, everyone deserves to be healthy and happy.

Q. Do you feel a beginner can access the feeling of the flow state either in yoga or surfing, or would you say it's more of an advanced practice that they can work their way up to with consistent dedicated practice?

A. The longer you practice yoga, the better it gets; same with surfing. You don't need to do it forever to get it, but know it just gets better. I've been practicing since I was eighteen. I'm thirty-five now, and people who know me say I've gotten more beautiful and emit a more brilliant energy than ever before. It's true: Human beings are meant to grow more beautiful with age. We're not meant to get old and ugly and full of disease. Yoga is a way to grow healthier, not only physically but mentally and energetically or spiritually, too. In yoga, you practice connecting to the spirit within you every day, and the more you practice, the stronger your connection. With time your energy grows, and more and more energy and inspiration flow through you. When you open up your mind and body to bring light into your world, it's like the spirit says, "Let's jump in this body and share love and wake everyone up!" It's a ride and it's not me doing it. It's me allowing the light to move through this mind and body I've been blessed with. When you realize you are neither your mind nor your body, your spirit can take over—then happiness comes. You must be contemplative though, and ask the spirit questions to allow insight to know what to do in any given moment.

I actually created a really powerful tool for this, called S.T.O.P. You use it when you need inspiration, whether when you feel upset and need to know how to deal with it, or if you just need inspiration for something fun too! The S stands for Stop, the T for Take a deep breath, the O for Observe, and the P for Perspective on peace and love. Violá, now write it down or put it in a pocket in your brain. Wear a bracelet to remind you to use it. Use it every day to create more peace and love in your life! Because isn't this what we all want? Here is a tool that can help you create what your spirit wants to move through you, love and light! So remember to Stop, Take a deep breath into your belly, Observe your mind and those around you, and gain Perspective on creating peace and love by asking, "What can I do to create more peace and love in this moment?" And then shift your perspective to one that creates peace and love. The answer may be to give a hug or a smile, go surfing, call a friend, do a meditation, or start a protest! This is how you connect with spirit, by opening yourself to be a pure vehicle for love in the world. Anyone can develop their consciousness; it's a matter of dedication and devotion.

Be aware that your mind will want to go back to suffering, but you can't let it. This is why you need to practice yoga. This is what being conscious means. You purify your being so you can live in a higher state of consciousness in celebration of who you are. Having a discipline to practice every day is the key. Without discipline, dedication, and reverence (bhakti), you cannot expect to get it. Write down what you want and what you can commit to every day to help you progress. Develop discipline, and you will be rewarded with more love and clarity!

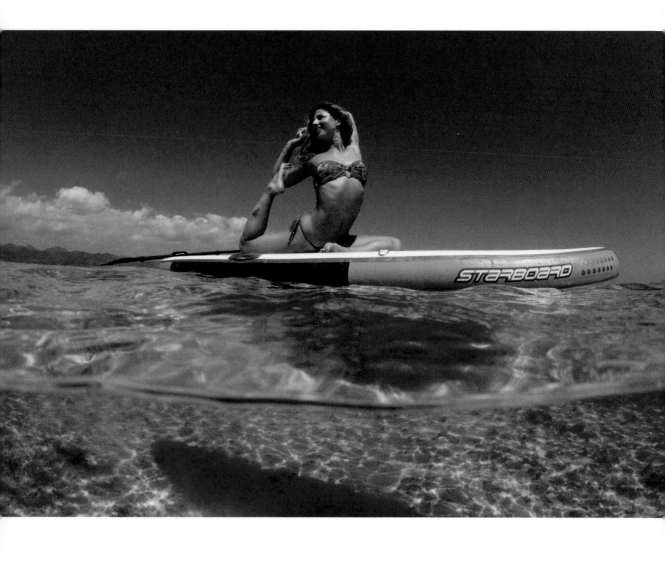

SUP YOGA MAGIC

Dashama Konah

I must be a mermaid . . . I have no fear of depths and a
great fear of shallow living.

—*Anaïs Nin*

SUP YOGA IS A PERFECT COMPLEMENT to the yoga and surfing
lifestyle. For the days when there are no waves, there's nothing better than going out on the ocean for a blissful yoga session to keep the
sacred connection between body, mind, and soul strong, while keeping
your energy clear and expansive. Even a few moments of SUP yoga can
completely wash away a stressful day and reset your mood and mindset.

Back in 2009 I was the first person to publish a video online demon-
strating this new innovation of yoga called SUP yoga. SUP stands for
stand-up paddling; I also wrote a chapter in the FalconGuide book *The
Art of Stand Up Paddling* if you'd like to learn more about this fun and
blissful water sport that's sweeping the planet and bringing joy to millions of people.

For me it was an obvious marriage between the two loves of my life:
yoga and the ocean. The experience of practicing yoga on a paddleboard, as opposed to on the beach or a yoga mat in a studio, is profound. There are both distinct and subtle differences in the practices,
and those who practice SUP yoga understand how these tiny distinc-
tions can be life changing in their effect on your mood, energy, yoga
practice, and overall outlook on life.

I feel that a chapter about SUP yoga belongs in this book since it is
somewhat a marriage of them both. Instead of practicing yoga on the

beach and then going out on the surfboard and riding the waves, we practice the asana on the board on the water. One of the principles I teach in my SUP yoga teacher trainings and retreats is called "grounding into the flow." In life where everything is constantly changing, which is exemplified by being on a board that is floating on top of the water in the ocean, a river, or a lake, for instance, we must learn to not only go with the flow, but to become "one with the flow."

That subtle difference may sound simple, but it is profound when you consider how hard it is for most people to simply go with the flow in life. I sometimes call going with the flow as being easygoing. It's a relationship to life that is in nonresistance to what is happening at any given moment. When we relax and accept life and "what is," exactly as it is, we can feel at peace and experience a sense of harmony within ourselves. That is essentially what all humans are seeking on some level. Whether they are aware of it or not, everyone on earth desires to be in harmony and to feel happy. Those are basic driving forces of life. Yet why are so few actually happy and feeling this sense of inner peace and well-being? The answer to this lies in the degree to which we are in resistance to what is, as opposed to simply being one with the flow of life, or as I call it, grounding into the flow.

It may sound contradictory at first: How can one be grounded when there is nothing solid to root down into? In the case of practicing yoga on a paddleboard, there appears to be a sense of solidness to the board itself, yet the water beneath it is in constant motion. Even on the calmest ocean, there is always a gentle current, as that is its very nature. Fluidity is never completely static, regardless of how still it may appear to the naked eye.

Life becomes much more enjoyable if we are not swimming against the stream all the time. When we are in resistance to the flow of life, we often run into major conflicts and challenges. This is a natural part of life, since humans do learn through pain, which can redirect us toward where we are supposed to be in life.

When we are out of alignment with our truth or have gotten off track from the highest and best course or path for our soul to achieve its purpose, we suffer. Maybe you can relate? Have you ever felt like you were in a pattern where many things were going wrong—perhaps your relationship was not in harmony, or financial matters were not in the flow? Did you stop to consider that perhaps these were all just signs redirecting you toward a destiny that is more aligned with your soul purpose? I invite you to consider this, as you go through this chapter, and the entire book. This insight alone can change the entire experience of your life if you are open to receive it on the deepest core level.

So how do you go about becoming grounded into the flow of life? Learning to truly listen to the voice within is an essential skill to master the art of living in the flow. If you tune in to how you are feeling, you can truly know what you should be doing, where you should be going, and who you should be with. It takes getting quiet inside and learning to listen to the voice within, which is always there like a loving friend to guide you in the right direction.

Every person we encounter and every experience are our teachers. We are being guided through these messages and messengers all along the journey, and if we have our eyes and ears tuned in to see and understand what these messages are, we can stay on course to achieve our destiny in life. That is what we are here for, to experience and learn all the blessings and lessons we need to grow, evolve, and expand toward our highest potential in this life.

Along this journey, we can choose to learn either through pain or joy. Both are great teachers. Let's choose to learn through joy! That is the very essence of SUP yoga—liberating yourself from the bonds of your mental, emotional, and physical obstructions, and in the process of letting them go, grounding into the ever-changing flow of life and connecting with the power of source, which is most alive and present when we are immersed in nature, breathing deeply, and doing what we love.

After teaching this blissful and powerful yoga-surf fusion for the past nine years, I have come to see we can learn so much from the physical practice of SUP yoga. As you embark upon this new adventure to take your yoga practice onto the paddleboard, I invite you to consider these philosophies while you experience each asana on the board.

Although you can practice almost any asana on the paddleboard, I have specifically chosen to share some of the more advanced practices to challenge you and to show you what is possible. Over the years I have had the opportunity to travel the world to some of the most pristine and exotic locations, such as Thailand, Japan, Indonesia, Hawaii, Bahamas, Spain, and even Germany, to spread the magic of this new and innovative yoga fusion. In partnership with my board sponsor, Starboard SUP (star-board.com), I've taught SUP yoga to children, grandparents, professional athletes, private clients, group classes, and events with over two hundred people on the water at once. We even developed a unique line of yoga paddleboards for my international Be the Change campaign to raise awareness about ocean conservation.

SUP yoga is not a trend or a fad; it's here to stay, just like yoga itself. As more people experience the profound effects it can have on your mood, energy, mindset, and overall perspective on life, I believe we will see yoga, surfing, and SUP yoga become even more widespread. These practices are not only for those elite athletes who have the courage to venture into the realms of the unknown and try something new. They are for everyone, and there is a starting place for all. Start where you are and learn the basics. As you build a solid foundation, you will begin to see the advancements you can experience in your overall consciousness, as each of these are profound and evolutionary paths that can lead to a liberation beyond your wildest imagination.

Have fun with it, and remember not to take anything in life too seriously. It is seriousness that makes us grow old. As we peel away the layers of all that we are not and leave these to be washed away in the vast loving waters of Mother Ocean, may we always remember the purpose for which we have come to live in this life. We each have a unique and powerful gift to offer to the world, unlike anyone else on earth, and it is our opportunity to discover what that is, to embrace it with all of our heart, and to share it with others as a way to make the world a better place from our presence here.

We can't take anything from this material world with us after we go, so let's enjoy the journey and leave a great impact that will be remembered for generations to come. The more you give and share, the more comes back to you, so share your gifts and your love freely with an open and compassionate heart. Tread lightly, as everything we do, each thought, action, and decision that we make, affects the world around us.

To paraphrase Gandhi, let's be the change we want to see in the world. The change starts with each of us. It's a simple choice. Start with yourself, start with self-love and self-care, be happy and spread goodness everywhere you go. Your life is a miracle. May you be blessed infinitely for the positive energy you put forth into the world. Let's all work together to make a difference here on earth. Join the movement, help clean up the beaches and the oceans, stop buying so much plastic, drive less, dance more, choose less conflict and more love.

8 SUP Yoga Poses + 5 Advanced Asanas for Inspiration

1. Lotus

For this seated meditation posture, you can try sukasana (easy pose), or if you have open hips, try the advanced option shown here, which is full lotus. For easy pose, simply sit in a comfortable cross-legged position, with spine straight and crown of the head lifted. A medium-difficulty option is to try half lotus, which will help to open your hip flexibility over time. For full lotus, start seated, bend your left knee, and draw the left foot in toward your right inner thigh. Then bend the right knee and place your right foot on top of the left thigh near your left hip crease. Keep both hips flat and lengthen the spine as you sit up straight and lift the crown of your head to the sky. Try to meditate here for a few moments, but be sure to come out of it if your knees start to feel any discomfort.

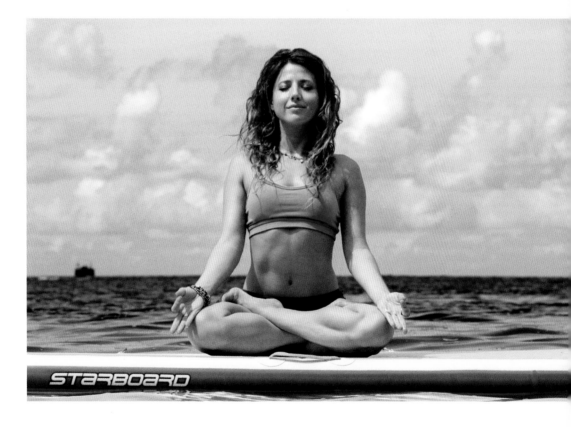

2. Side Plank

Start by lying on your right side with legs straight and right hand placed beneath the right shoulder. Side plank on a paddleboard is a lot more challenging than on land. There are some modifications you can start with that may help. Try using the top leg to stabilize by either bending the knee and placing the foot in front of the bottom leg or at least staggering the feet so they are heel to toe to create a wider foundation at the base of this pose. You can also keep your elbow bent and balance on your forearm to start, and then try to extend the arm fully into side plank when you feel stable. Using core stability will help here tremendously. Lift your hips and, if possible, extend the upper arm either toward the sky or over the top ear to lengthen the side body. Hold for 3–5 breaths and repeat on the other side.

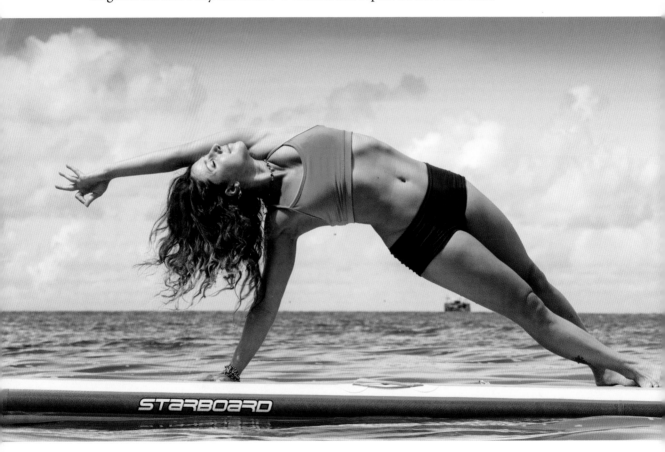

3. Camel

For this heart-opening backbend, start kneeling with feet, shins, and knees hip-distance apart. Tuck your tailbone under as you lengthen your spine from the lower lumbar, lifting your heart toward the sky as you place your hands on your ankles and gently arch back. If your neck feels open, feel free to lay your head back and look back. If your spine isn't flexible enough to reach both ankles yet, tuck your toes under to raise the heels and ankles closer to your hands, and then place your hands on your ankles. Hold for a few breaths, and be sure to come back into child's pose to counter the backbend with a forward bend.

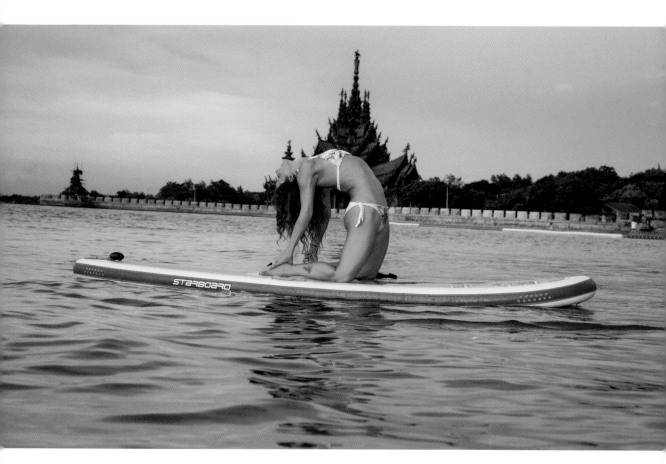

4. Down Dog

This is one of the most stable poses you can do on the board. With both hands and feet firmly rooted onto the board, be sure to position yourself directly in the center; the wider you place your hands and feet, the stabler you will feel. As you root down through the palms, with fingers spread wide, lengthen your spine, lift your tailbone toward the sky, and press your chest in toward your thighs. Hold for 3–5 breaths and then lower to your hands and knees. Repeat 3 times or go through a vinyasa series with up dog and plank to transition. This pose strengthens your entire body while opening the upper back, shoulders, calves, and hamstrings.

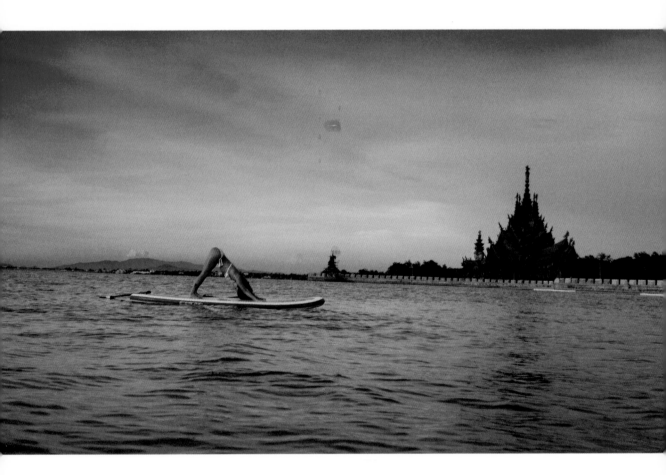

5. Crescent Lunge

Start in a low lunge with your right foot forward, right knee at a 90-degree angle, and left leg extended back behind you with the knee on the board and the top of the foot planted firmly to stabilize. Engage your core and squeeze your thighs toward each other to hug the midline and stabilize. First option is to keep your hands on the board on either side of your front foot. Second option is to place one hand on the board and raise the other hand and arm toward the sky. Third option is to reach both arms up and above your head. Palms can be in prayer, or interlace the fingers to feel more centered. Radiate your hips forward and lift your heart to the sky. Hold for 3–5 breaths and repeat on the other side.

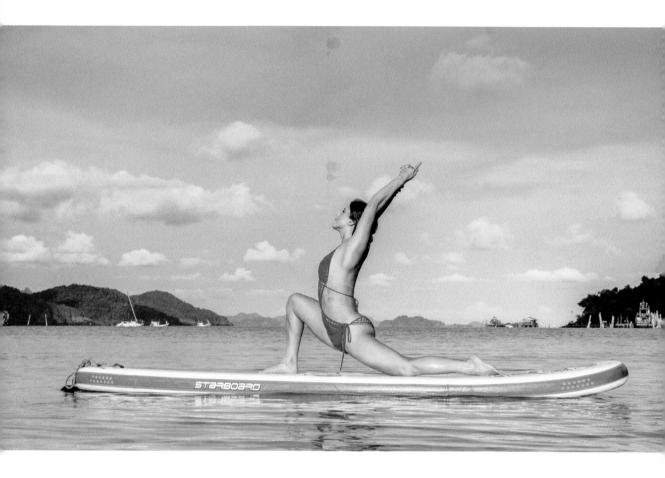

6. Triangle

Start standing on the board with the right foot forward and the left foot back, back foot perpendicular to the front arch so you have a firm foundation. Root down through the soles of your feet to create a bandha, or energy lock, to keep you grounded. Placing your right hand on the foot, ankle, or inside of the foot on the board, extend the top arm up toward the sky. Drishti, or gaze, is up toward the top hand, or you can gaze to the side or down if that helps you to stabilize. Use your core strength and mula bandha (root lock), hips spread wide, and lengthen the spine and front knee. Take 3–5 deep breaths.

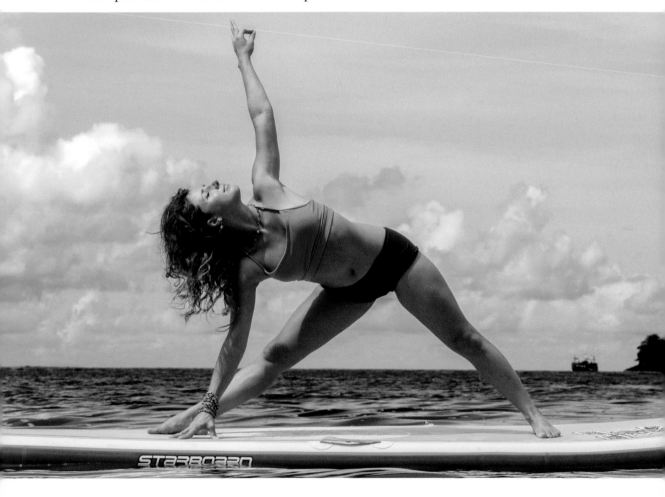

7. Warrior 2

This is a challenging, powerful standing pose that requires great stability and focus. Start the same as triangle with your right foot forward and left foot back and strong foundation positioning. Bend the front knee to a 90-degree angle, being sure to not overextend the knee in front of the ankle. Engage your core and tuck the tailbone slightly to lengthen your spine, engage your bandhas to lock your energy in, and, if it helps, angle your front foot in slightly as you hug the midline of your body between the points of the front knee and back hip to stabilize even more. Lift your chest and extend your arms out in both directions, reaching forward and back, gazing forward past your front fingertips. Hold for a few breaths and slowly transition to repeat the same pose on the other side.

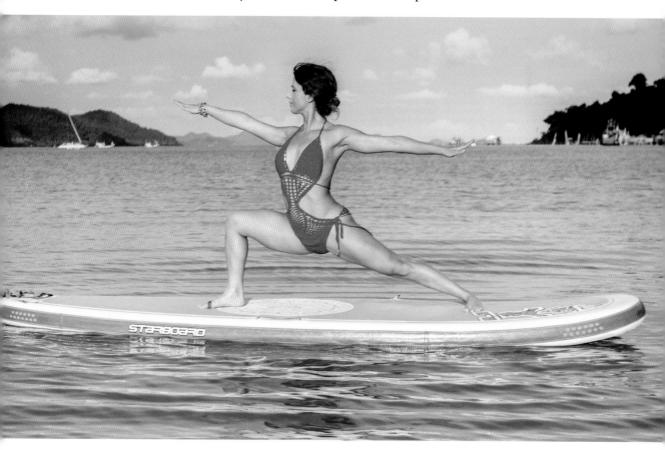

8. Splits

This is an advanced pose, so if you don't yet have the flexibility, you can start with half splits. Starting in a low lunge with your left foot forward and right knee back, straighten the front leg as you fold forward over that leg. Stabilize by grounding down through both palms on the board on either side of the front foot. If you can reach your left hand to your left foot, pull your toes back toward your face as you lengthen your spine and hamstrings. Take 3–5 breaths and repeat on the other side. If you can extend all the way down into full splits, slide the back leg back and front leg forward until you can sit comfortably in splits (hanumanasana). This pose is at once grounding, opening, and challenging. Breathe deeply and be sure to do both sides.

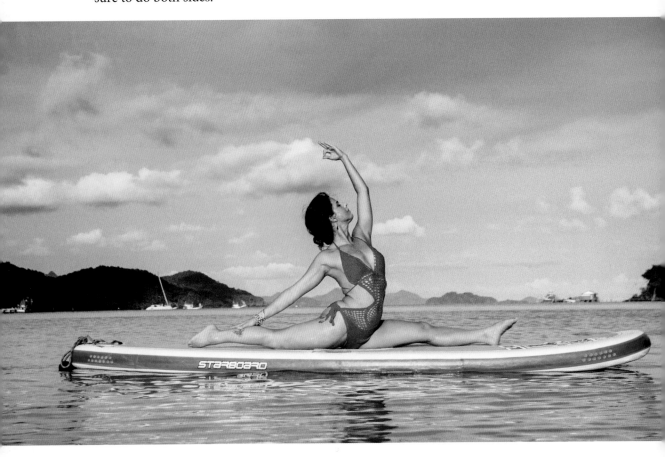

These last five asanas are advanced poses that require great strength, balance, and flexibility. I suggest you master these on land before trying them on the board. Use these images as inspiration for what is possible, and work toward each one by increasing your balance, strength, and flexibility over time.

9. Scorpion

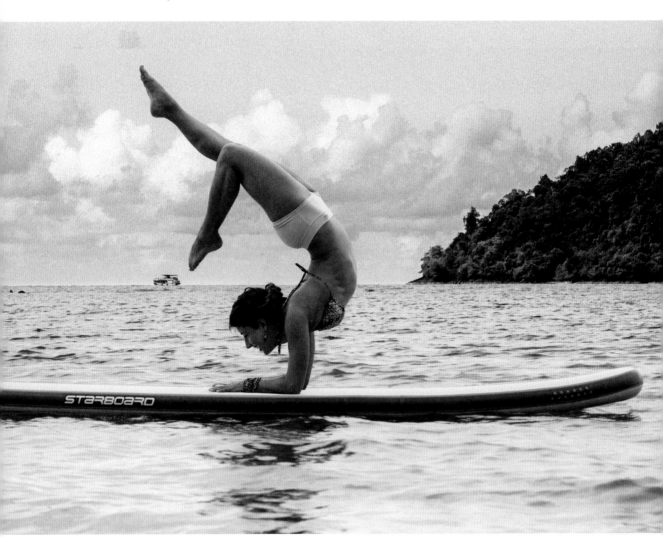

10. Leg Behind Head Arm Balance

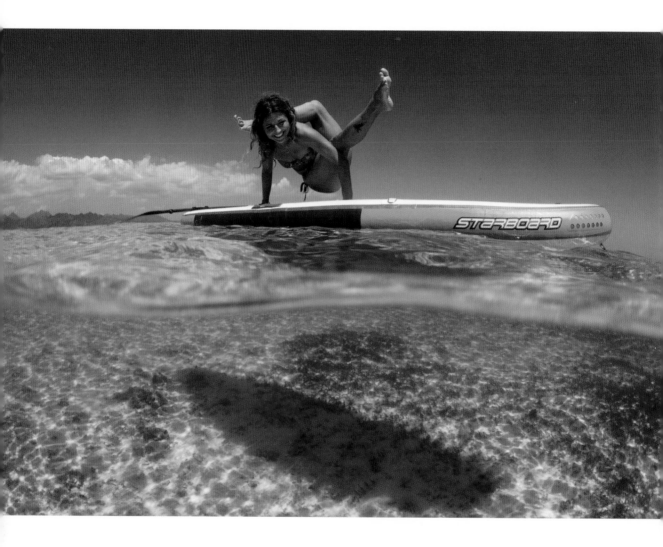

11. Locust

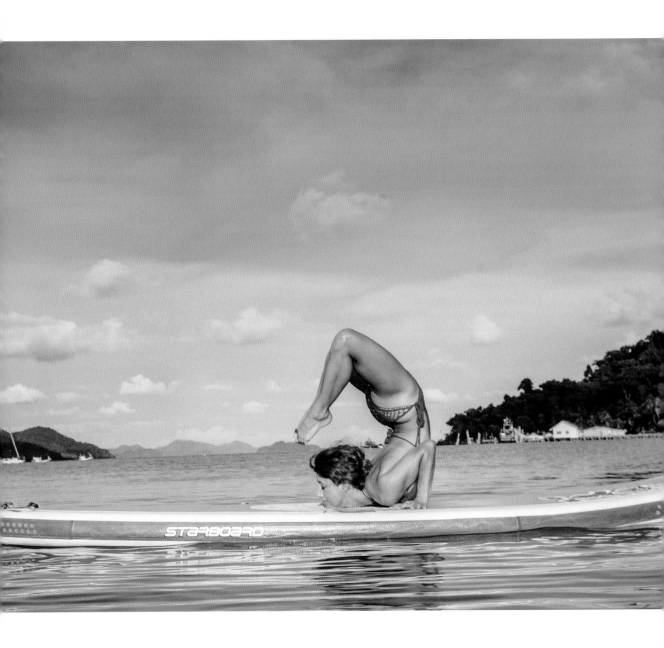

12. Hollow Back Wheel

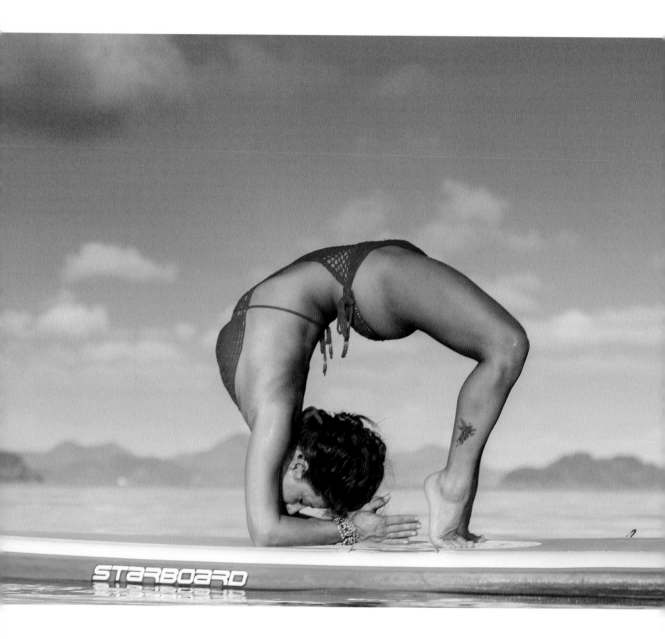

13. King Pigeon

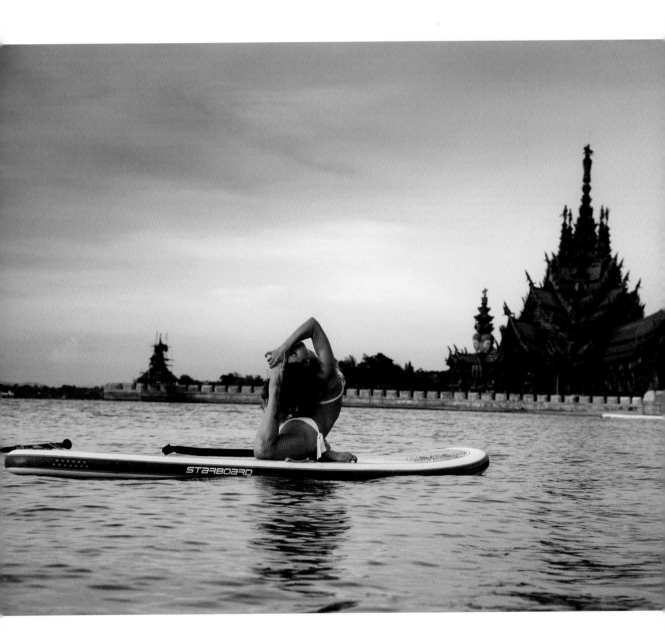

About Dashama's SUP Yoga

Dashama is an international SUP yoga athlete and yoga teacher who leads SUP yoga teacher trainings, retreats, and events worldwide. Credited as the original innovator in the field of SUP yoga, she published the first SUP yoga video online in 2009 and began teaching this new fusion yoga style at the Waldorf Astoria Resort in Boca Raton, Florida. She is the global yoga ambassador for Starboard SUP, one of the top-selling paddleboard and water sports manufacturers in the world, whose brand is based on environmental sustainability, innovation, and quality. She has collaborated with Starboard to create the Dashama Astro line of travel-friendly yoga boards and has traveled extensively with the international team of board riders for PR events, media appearances, photo and video shoots, and to teach SUP yoga in Germany, Spain, Tokyo, Thailand, Indonesia, Hawaii, and Miami. To learn more about the Dashama Astro inflatable yoga paddle-boards, visit sup-yoga.com; to learn about upcoming SUP yoga trainings and retreats, visit Dashama's website at dashama.com.

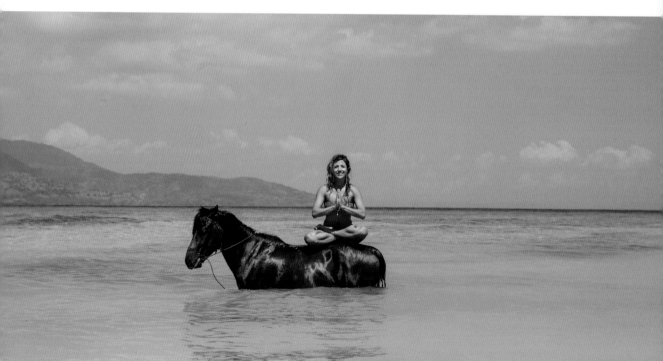

AFTERWORD

MAHALO. Thank you for taking the time to explore *Yoga for Surfing* with us.

As you can see, there are a variety of ways and expressions in which yoga and surfing are being practiced, shared, and experienced. There is never only one way, and all ways are equally powerful and valid. As you embark upon this path and journey toward experiencing the flow state through yoga and surfing, I invite you to keep an open heart and mind. Look for the messages and messengers throughout your journey, and remain grateful for the miracle of life.

Thousands of years of human experience has brought yoga to the forefront of modern medicine as a proven path to prevent, heal, and cure sickness, disease, and most ailments that are rooted in what is often called "stress." Stress is simply being out of harmony with yourself, your soul, and the source of life. Through my partnership with Harvard and Warwick University, I have embarked upon a research program to validate and explore yoga's positive effect on human well-being in the corporate setting, as that affects the vast majority of individuals in modern society who work in offices and live in urban areas.

As we expand our reach through yoga into the farthest corners of humanity and the world, we discover more ways to share this ancient and powerful practice, science, art, and system of conscious evolution. I invite you to take your practice deeper if you should feel called, by connecting with me or any of the teachers or masters who have contributed to make this book possible. Find who resonates with you and reach out to us. Let us know where you are on the path and how we can help make your journey more meaningful and deepen your understanding of yoga or surfing.

All the contributors in this book have included their bio with links to their websites along with the best ways to keep in touch. As an added bonus, feel free to visit my websites at dashama.com or pranashama.com to access free yoga videos, audios, and ebooks to take your practice to the next level. You can also join our team to help raise awareness about ocean conservation through our initiative with this book. Together as a global tribe we aim to eradicate the pollution, contamination, and destruction of the ocean, which represents over 70 percent of the earth's surface and provides us with over 50 percent of the oxygen we need to breathe and stay alive. Together with our partners at Surfrider Foundation and Virgin Ocean Unite, we are hosting local, national, and global events, gatherings, and initiatives to create opportunities for you to be involved. There are many ways you can help, and together we can all achieve more. Donate your time, money, and resources; spread the word and take a stand for what you believe in. Every little thing you do affects everything else. We are all part of the grand fabric of life, and we are here to learn, grow, connect, and experience this life in all the magical and miraculous ways we can.

Consider joining us at a retreat, event, or teacher training in paradise, and remember, you always have a family with us, wherever you are. We are connected by the One Source of Life that created us all. Keep diving deep, surfing the crests of the waves of life, and staying in the flow.

Many blessings to you on the path.

Love and Namaste,
Dashama

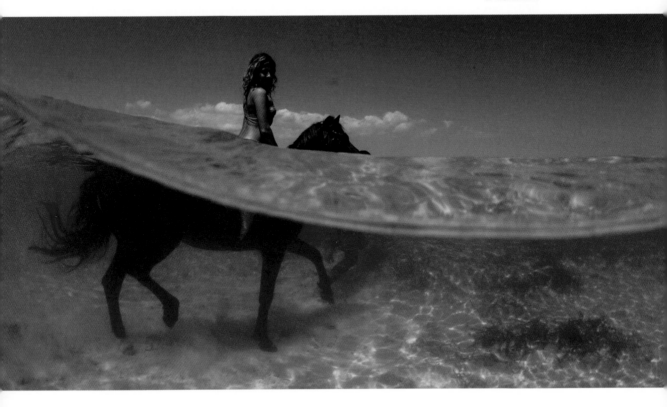

PHOTO CREDITS

Photos on pp. i, iv, vi, ix, and 200 by Mick Curley with Starboard SUP

Chapter 1: Beach Yoga Bliss
All photos by Irina Kazakova, Bahamas, except on p. 2 (by Dashama Konah) and p. 19 (Mick Curley with Starboard SUP)

Chapter 2: Embody the Flow
All photos by Shiva Rea, Yoga Adventures

Chapter 3: Yoga for Surfers Pioneer
All photos by David Hall

Chapter 4: Blissology
All photos by Carin Smolinski except on p. 55 (by Olivia Nachle), p. 59 (by Damea Dorsey), and p. 65 (by Ali Kaukas)

Chapter 5: Swell Living
All photos by Abe Shouse, Starshot Media, Big Island, Hawaii

Chapter 6: Born to Surf
All photos by Zane Schweitzer

Chapter 7: Yogi Surfing Ocean Mamma
All photos by Luz Castillo Zarco

Chapter 8: SUP Surf Yoga
All photos by Marissa Williams

Chapter 9: Yoga for Happiness
All photos by Jianca Lazarus except on pp. 138 and 142 (by Lulu Dropo, Oahu, Hawaii); p. 140 (by Juan Cabanas); p. 143 (by Jianca Lazarus); p. 151 (by Aaron Mizushima)

Chapter 10: Guru Yoga for Surfers
All photos by Joe Lyman

Chapter 11: SUP Yoga Magic
All photos by Mick Curley with Starboard SUP

INDEX

ABOUT THE AUTHOR

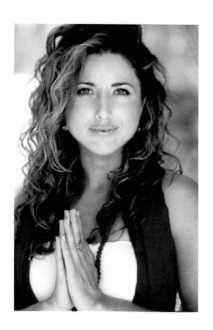

Dashama is a yoga, health, and happiness expert with books, DVDs, and online training programs distributed worldwide. She is the founder of Pranashama Yoga Institute, which leads yoga teacher trainings and retreats globally. An innovator in the field of yoga, as a result of her love of the ocean through surfing and paddleboarding, she created the fusion water sport known globally know as SUP yoga or paddleboard yoga. She has been featured worldwide on magazine covers, newspaper articles, TV news, and online media as an expert, athlete, teacher, and innovator.